GRAY-SCALE ULTRASOUND:

A Manual for Physicians and Technical Personnel

ROYAL J. BARTRUM, JR., M.D.   **HARTE C. CROW, M.D.**

Department of Diagnostic Radiology
Hitchcock Clinic
Dartmouth Medical School
Hanover, New Hampshire

1977
W. B. SAUNDERS COMPANY
Philadelphia, London, Toronto

W. B. Saunders Company: West Washington Square
Philadelphia, PA 19105

1 St. Anne's Road
Eastbourne, East Sussex BN21 3UN, England

1 Goldthorne Avenue
Toronto, Ontario M8Z 5T9, Canada

Gray-Scale Ultrasound: A Manual for Physicians and Technical Personnel   ISBN   0-7216-1548-1

Last digit is the print number: 9   8   7   6   5   4   3   2   1

To Sheila, Jane, and Ann.

PREFACE

Diagnostic ultrasound has come of age. In late 1973 abdominal and pelvic ultrasound was considered an interesting new imaging modality, but its use was confined to scattered medical centers throughout the world. At that time the number of technicians and physicians doing ultrasound was so small that literally "everybody knew everyone else," and information on technical and clinical developments circulated informally. There were no textbooks on the subject, no postgraduate courses, a single fledgling journal, a small and widely scattered literature, and only three hospitals in the United States offering any formal training in the field.

Then, in late 1974, gray-scale ultrasound scanners became commercially available. For the first time images looked like pictures instead of Rorschach ink blots. Physician interest was awakened. At the same time CT X-ray scanners dramatically proved the value of cross-sectional imaging. Ultrasound scanning was accepted as a vital part of the diagnostic armamentarium, something which should be available in the community hospital as well as the medical center.

This unprecedented demand for ultrasound services has revealed a dramatic shortage of training facilities for the continually increasing numbers of physicians and technologists involved in ultrasound. Several texts on scanning have been published and have helped fill this need. Unfortunately, most of these volumes were conceived and written during the era of bi-stable scanning and could not anticipate the rapid technologic equipment advances which have occurred. Also these texts are directed toward interpretation of ultrasound images and provide little information on the technique of producing scans of good quality. Postgraduate courses abound, but these also concentrate on image interpretation rather than image production. There are some in-residence "fellowship" training programs, but spaces are limited; and these programs cannot absorb the numbers of physicians and technologists entering the field.

In order to establish adequate standards for technicians in ultrasound the Registry of Diagnostic Medical Sonographers was established in 1975 and conducted the first qualifying examinations in June, 1976. Both a written and practical examination were required of candidates. We had the privilege of conducting some of these examinations and the results were distressing. While many of the candidates were highly knowledgeable and excellent sonographers, there was a large number who were insufficiently prepared to conduct a diagnostic examination of quality. All of the candidates expressed frustration at having no source for information and training in scanning. Most said that the physicians for whom they worked could not provide this information, as they themselves could not perform the examination from a technical standpoint.

v

Physicians seem frustrated by the same shortage of basic instruction material. For over two years we have offered a one- or two-week postgraduate fellowship for physicians in B-mode ultrasound. This course was designed for the community radiologist who had just acquired an ultrasound machine but didn't know how to turn it on. To make matters worse, he was often too busy with his practice to take off three or six months to travel some distance to take an intensive course on the subject. Sometimes he sent his favorite technician to a course instead, or tried to hire an experienced technician away from some-place else. This usually backfired: the favorite technician either came back poorly trained or, if well-trained, was quickly hired away by some other desperate physician. Perhaps even more frustrating were the situations in which the untrained physician was at the mercy of the well-trained tech-nologist—although the physician signed the reports, his signature was mean-ingless because the technician actually performed and interpreted the exam-ination. What we tried to offer in our brief two weeks was a firm footing in the realm of B-mode scanning; although our "graduates" did not leave as ultra-sound experts, they left with enough knowledge to judge the technical merits of an ultrasound scan and even perform a credible examination themselves. They were equipped to continue to learn and expand their ultrasound knowl-edge. Well, things went nicely at first—just a few fellows now and then, but not enough to interfere seriously with our normal routine or disrupt our resi-dent teaching. But business just kept on improving. Despite the fact that we did not advertise the fellowship, did not have a "glamour" name, and were located out in the boonies of New Hampshire, the demand for the fellowship outstripped our ability to provide it. Since we do not have a monopoly on ultrasound teaching, we assume this trend indicates an ever-increasing de-mand for basic B-mode ultrasound instruction.

It is these experiences which have motivated us to produce this book. Abdominal and pelvic ultrasonography is the most demanding of any imaging modality. In contrast to CT and radioisotope scanning, in which technician input is small, or conventional radiography for which most technical factors can be standardized, ultrasound image quality (and consequent diagnostic accuracy) is totally dependent upon the skill of the machine operator, be it technician or physician. It is obvious that unless both the technician and the physician involved in ultrasound are capable of producing high quality, re-producible scans which are free of artifacts, there is little value in establishing an ultrasound service.

This book is, therefore, directed to all those who are new to ultrasound scanning of the abdomen and pelvis and who plan to work in these areas. It discusses the many factors involved in organizing an ultrasound laboratory and generating scans of useful diagnostic quality. The material is rather dogmatic. This is by design. We certainly do not pretend that our way of scanning is the only way or necessarily the best way; in ultrasound, as any endeavor, "there is more than one way to skin a cat." We do know, however, that the techniques and methods described work for us and that they will work for others. We feel it is important for anyone beginning scanning to have a firm basis upon which to expand and experiment. Once the methods in this book are mastered, the ultrasonographer should continually modify and expand his technique until he evolves a method which works best for him.

There is little discussion of scan interpretation; other texts and journals cover this topic nicely and our bibliography lists some of these sources of information. The most difficult part of interpreting ultrasound scans is producing a technically adequate image and deciding what is real and what is artifact: we cover that problem in detail.

Similarly, there is little discussion of bi-stable scanning. Although still an extremely important adjuvant to many examinations, the general utility of bi-stable scanners is limited. Modern ultrasound is gray-scale ultrasound.

We have included a chapter on the technique of ultrasonically guided biopsy. Although not yet a widely used procedure, this exciting aspect of ultrasound has the potential for extending dramatically the medical diagnostic process.

Finally a brief word about style. It will quickly become apparent that we have abandoned the traditional medical discourse and substituted informal discussion. Although it may offend some readers we have chosen to do this for two reasons. First, we have written this book not only for the physician but also for the technician, medical student, and medical voyeur. To encompass this disparity of backgrounds, we have tried to avoid jargon and simplify explanations insofar as possible. Second, throughout our schooling we were "lectured at" and subtly resented it. We are all adults now: it is time to discuss things as partners rather than as masters and pupils.

But enough procrastination — off to the ultrasound lab!

ROYAL J. BARTRUM, JR.

HARTE C. CROW

ACKNOWLEDGMENTS

Any book is like an iceberg. The authors represent the tip; supporting them is a large group of unseen collaborators. We would like to note the following:

First and foremost, Sheila R. Foote, R.T., ultrasonographer extraordinaire and chief ultrasound technician at the Dartmouth-Hitchcock Medical Center. Coming from Groveton, New Hampshire (you have to see it to believe it), and starting with no ultrasound knowledge whatever, she is an inspiring example of how common sense, experience and dedication can lead to genuine expertise in scanning.

Our other ultrasound technicians, Carol Bailey, R.T., Kathy Horan, R.T., and Marty Keyes, R.T., have also provided both technical and moral support throughout this project.

Many trusting and patient folks consented to be models for scanning, among them Joyce Cilley, Donald Chakares, Laura Jo Helff, Patricia Huke, Martha McDaniel, Gerard Smith, and Cindy Watson.

Valarie Page contributed the lucid diagrams which help unscramble our prose.

Betsy Youngholm and Linda Rondeau converted our hen-scratchings and garbled dictation to legible typescript.

Finally, George Vilk, of W. B. Saunders Company, provided considerable encouragement while showing uncommon patience at our continually late manuscripts.

To all, our heartfelt thanks.

R.J.B.

H.C.C.

CONTENTS

Chapter 1

PRACTICAL PHYSICS

Do not skip this chapter! We hate physics just as much as you do, probably more. It would be wonderful if ultrasound scanners were totally standardized and automated so that all that was required to produce an image was simply to place the patient in front of the machine, push a button, and develop a picture. Alas, this is not the case at the present time. There is no field of medical imaging that is more dependent upon the skill of the machine operator than ultrasound scanning. And it is impossible to become a competent machine operator unless you know something about how the machine works.

We do not mean that you have to know enough physics to tear the scanner apart and rebuild the insides using leftover color TV parts, bubble gum, and a bobby pin; or that you have to be able to crystallize your own transducers on the kitchen stove. We mean only that you must have a basic understanding of what the ultrasound beam is, why an echo is produced, why artifacts exist, and what the various knobs on the machine do to the picture and why.

This is similar to the knowledge you must have to operate any mechanical contrivance adequately. The automobile is a good example. Most of us are not mechanics and don't know a piston from a pushrod or preignition from a marble in the ashtray, yet we do know a fair amount about the practical physics of the car. For instance, we know that gasoline is burned in the engine and produces energy to run the rest of the car. We know that this process is started by another form of energy, electricity in the battery, which runs the starter. Therefore if we turn the key and nothing happens we are more likely to suspect that the battery is dead rather than that the car is out of gas. Knowing this, we would ask someone to give us a push start rather than set off down the road, gas can in hand. Similarly if we were driving along and the car stopped, we would think the problem was more likely to be an empty gas tank than a dead battery.

It is this same general level of knowledge of the practical physics of ultrasound image production that is required. That is what this chapter is about—the physics of ultrasound for those who hate physics. We wish we could have put it at the end of the book—we know it is a bummer and a terrible lead-off topic, but unfortunately it is the basic platform upon which all ultrasound scanning rests and you simply must understand some of it before any other aspect of scanning will make much sense.

Enough procrastination. Getting into physics is like getting into an ice-cold swimming pool; the only way to do it is to hold your nose and jump.

THE PULSE-ECHO PRINCIPLE

B-mode ultrasonography is based on the pulse-echo principle. (We are going to discuss the term "B-mode" at some length later; for the moment it is enough to say that this term is a way of describing the information display system used almost exclusively in ultrasound scanning of any part of the body except the heart.)

A man stands on one side of a canyon and shouts "Hello!" toward the other side. This is the "pulse." That pulse travels through the air at the speed of sound (about 741 miles an hour) until it hits the opposite wall of the canyon where it is reflected back toward the man. Once the pulse has been reflected it becomes an "echo." The echo travels back to the man at the same speed of sound and, after a brief period of time, he hears the echo. We have all participated in this type of pulse-echo experience.

If the man has a stopwatch (and a small electronic calculator) he can use this pulse-echo to calculate how far it is to the other side of the canyon. He simply measures the time it took for his shout (the pulse) to be echoed back to him. Suppose this was 4 seconds. He consults his handy conversion table which tells him that 741 miles per hour is equivalent to 1087 feet per second. He then multiplies 1087 feet per second by 4 seconds and discovers that his "Hello" traveled 4348 feet. Since this represented two trips across the canyon (one for the pulse going and the other for the echo returning) he then divides by 2 and obtains 2174 feet as the distance to the other side of the canyon.

Now if the man got a kick out of measuring canyons this way, he would probably get tired of doing all these calculations every time he 'shouted. Instead he would sit down with a six-pack and do all of the calculations once for every possible time from 1 to, say, 20 seconds. He would then repaint the face of his stopwatch so that, instead of reading in seconds, it would read the number of feet to the echo source. Then he would be all set to measure canyons easily and quickly, using only his shout and the calibrated watch. Of course, his calibrated watch would be accurate only as long as the speed of sound was 1087 feet per second, but since the speed of sound in air doesn't vary much, at least when compared to the accuracy with which he can read his stopwatch, this problem isn't of much concern.

ULTRASOUND

Ultrasound imaging uses this same pulse-echo principle. A short pulse of ultrasound is emitted into the body. This pulse travels through the tissues at a constant speed until it encounters a reflecting surface. At such a surface some of the sound beam is reflected back toward the source; there it is received by the ultrasound scanner, which has been keeping track of the time and converting it to a distance in the same manner as the man and his calibrated stopwatch. However, instead of giving out the distance as a number, the

scanner shows it as a dot or a spike on an oscilloscope or TV screen; the position of the spike is proportional to the distance the echo traveled. This enables us not only to measure the distance but to get a visual picture of it as well.

Although the principle of ultrasonic pulse-echo diagnosis is the same as the echo in the canyon there are several practical differences. To understand these differences we need to know a little about sound.

All sound, be it ultrasound or the kind we hear, is actually a series of repeating pressure waves. It is convenient to think about these waves and illustrate them as sine wave forms, as shown in Figure 1–1. Line A shows a single wave or cycle. As we move along the horizontal axis, which represents time, the pressure starts at zero, rises to some peak, then falls back to zero and continues to a negative value before returning to zero. Line B shows a continuous wave form where a large number of the single waves have been strung together. The single wave is analogous to an extremely short beep of a car horn while the continuous wave represents the horn being stuck in the on position.

This simple wave form is not adequate to fully describe the sound, however. We must know more information about the

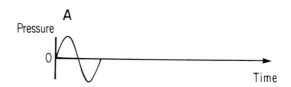

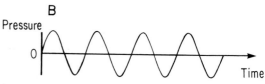

Figure 1–1. A diagrammatic representation of sound as a sine wave. A, A single wave or cycle. The horizontal axis is time; the vertical axis is pressure at a point in the medium through which the sound is traveling. The wave starts at zero pressure, rises to some positive value, then falls past zero to a negative value before returning to its starting position.

B, A continuous sound wave, made up of several single cycles linked together.

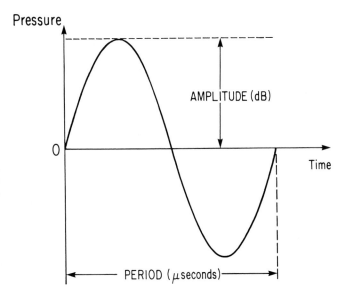

Figure 1-2. Some of the common parameters of a sound beam and the units in which they are commonly expressed.

VELOCITY (meters/sec) = Speed of sound (~1540 meters/second for human soft tissue)

FREQUENCY (MHz) = 1/PERIOD

WAVELENGTH (millimeters) = VELOCITY/FREQUENCY

wave before we can predict how it will behave. Therefore, several pieces of data are described for these waves (such data are called parameters of the wave). Some of the more important parameters are illustrated in Figure 1-2. The **period** is the time it takes to complete a single cycle. The **amplitude** is the peak pressure or height of the wave. This is a measure of the strength or "loudness" of the sound wave. A shouted "Hello" has a large amplitude while a whispered "Hello" has a small amplitude. We will use the words "power," "intensity," and "loudness" interchangeably with amplitude. While, in a strict physical sense, each of these terms has a slightly different meaning, for our purposes it will cause no errors to think of them as describing the same quantity.

The **velocity** is the speed of the wave. The velocity depends on the type of material in which the wave is traveling. For instance, in air sound travels 741 miles per hour, which is equivalent to 331 meters per second (from here on we will use the metric system for all measurements). In stainless steel sound travels at 3100 meters per second. And in human soft tissue at 37° Centigrade (body temperature) sound travels at 1540 meters per second.

The **frequency** is the number of times the wave is repeated per second. The frequency is calculated by dividing the period (the time it takes to complete a single cycle) into 1.

Finally there is the **wavelength,** which is the distance the wave travels during a single cycle. The wavelength is calculated by dividing the velocity by the frequency.

Fortunately we will not have to be concerned with making all these calculations since only a very few different frequencies and wavelengths are used in ultrasound and it is easy to remember them.

Now we can see how ultrasound differs from the sound we hear. First, and most important, is frequency. Audible sound ranges in frequency from 16 to 20,000 cycles per second (a cycle per second is known as a Hertz; a million cycles per second is called a MegaHertz and is abbreviated MHz). Ultrasound is defined as any sound with a frequency of greater than 20,000 Hertz. In abdominal B-scanning we use sound frequencies ranging from 1 to 5 MHz.

The next consideration is velocity. Although velocity is independent of frequency and is determined by the medium in which the sound is traveling, there are practical differences. Since we hear sound in air, the velocity of audible sound is 331 meters per second. However, we use ultrasound in human soft tissue so the velocity in which we are interested is 1540 meters per second. (This is an average value; the actual velocities vary slightly from tissue to tissue, but these differences are so small that we can use the average value and not introduce any serious errors.)

The wavelengths of audible sound range from 2 to 200 centimeters while the wavelengths used in B-mode ultrasound range from 0.3 to 1.5 millimeters. (A millimeter is 1/10 of a centimeter; a Virginia Slims cigarette is 120 millimeters long.)

The amplitude or power of the ultrasound used for diagnosis is much smaller than that needed to shout "Hello." Since amplitudes vary so widely and since, for most purposes, we are not as concerned with the actual amplitude as with the relationship of one amplitude to another, a different type of measure of amplitude is used for sound. This is the decibel (dB) notation which is based on comparing the amplitudes of two different sound waves. We are all familiar with this type of measurement and use it every day. For example, in describing the virtues of a football quarterback we might say that quarterback A can throw the ball *twice as far* as quarterback B; or we say that a Mack truck weighs *ten times as much* as a Volkswagen. In neither case do we talk about the actual number of feet the football is thrown or the number of pounds the truck weighs. Of course, if we have in our mind some concept of how much a Volkswagen weighs (perhaps from tipping one over in our younger days) we could describe other vehicles in terms of how they compare to a Volkswagen and, at the same time, have some idea of their actual weight as well. In this sense a comparative measurement system can be used as if the numbers corresponded to some real quantity. Even though it is not really correct to use decibels as if they were some real and absolute measure of sound amplitude or power, it is useful and convenient to do so and will not introduce any errors into our thinking. So, we will often refer to

the amplitude of ultrasound echoes as X number of decibels: the greater the number of decibels, the greater the amplitude (or the "louder") the echo.

Before we leave this topic of decibels, we should point out that this is a logarithmic system; that is, a decibel is defined as: $dB = 20 \log \frac{E_2}{E_1}$; where E_2 and E_1 are the actual measurements of the amplitudes of two different echoes.* Logarithmic scales are used whenever the quantities involved cover very large ranges; this enables widely different numbers to be easily compared. You have probably noticed already that 20 decibels corresponds to a factor of 10. Thus if echo A is 20 decibels louder than echo B, echo A has 10 *times* the amplitude of echo B. In a typical abdominal or pelvic ultrasound scan the echoes received from the soft tissues range in strength from 0 to 60 decibels. The actual amplitude range of these echoes is therefore 1 to 1000. (You have probably also figured out that quarterback A is 6 dB better than quarterback B and that a Mack truck is 20 dB heavier than a Volkswagen.)

INTERACTION OF ULTRASOUND AND TISSUE

Sound traveling through air, such as the "Hello" of our friend, the canyon measurer, has a pretty uncomplicated life. It simply zips across the canyon, hits the far wall, and comes rebounding back. About the only really noticeable change is that the sound gets weaker as it travels, so the echo is not nearly as loud as the shout. When an ultrasonic pulse is sent into the soft tissues of the body, however, it undergoes continuous modification.

The most significant change is attenuation. Although not a scientifically rigorous definition, we shall consider **attenuation** to be the progressive weakening of the sound beam as it travels through tissue. Thus, the farther through the tissue the sound travels,

---

*This definition of the decibel is used when electric power is involved, and since echoes produce electric signals, this is the definition used in diagnostic ultrasound. For other purposes the decibel is defined as: $dB = 10 \log \frac{P_2}{P_1}$.

the weaker it gets. The attenuation of ultrasound is dependent on many factors, including the wavelength of the sound, the type and density of the tissue, the degree of heterogeneity of the tissue, and the number and type of echo interfaces in the tissue. It is impossible to predict accurately the degree of attenuation for something as complex as human tissue. Nevertheless, it is no great problem to measure the attenuation in a laboratory (the amplitude of the sound beam is measured at varying distances in a tissue and the difference, after some mathematical manipulation, becomes the attenuation).

Attenuation measurements have been made for many different human tissues with many different frequencies of ultrasound. These figures are available in textbooks on the physics of ultrasound. The actual numbers are of no great concern to the average clinical ultrasonographer, but it is useful to remember the following general rule of thumb: the "average" attenuation of an ultrasound beam in human soft tissue is 1 dB per centimeter per MHz. This means that an ultrasound beam with a frequency of 1 MHz loses 1 dB of amplitude for every centimeter it travels. A 2.25 MHz beam loses $2.25 \times 1 = 2.25$ dB for every centimeter it travels and a 5 MHz beam loses $5 \times 1 = 5$ dB per centimeter. We must remember that each echo received has actually traveled *twice* as far as the distance to the reflecting surface since it has made a trip to the reflecting surface and back to the source. Therefore, we must multiply the attenuation by 2 if we wish to know how much an echo from any given depth has been attenuated.

(Just to make sure we all have this straight before going on, we will now have a short quiz. *The question:* "An ultrasound beam with a frequency of 3.5 MHz is directed into the liver and an echo is received from a depth of 6 centimeters. How much has this echo been attenuated?" *The answer:* "Attenuation is estimated as 1 dB per centimeter per MHz. 1 dB × 3.5 MHz = 3.5 dB per centimeter. The echo came from 6 centimeters but it actually traveled 12 centimeters—6 going out and 6 coming back—so we multiply 3.5 dB per centimeter × 12 centimeters = 42 dB. The echo was attenuated by 42 dB.")

How does attenuation of an ultrasound beam occur? Primarily through three processes: absorption, reflection, and scattering.

Absorption occurs when energy in the sound beam is captured (or absorbed) by the tissue. Most of this energy is converted to heat in the tissue. It is this process which is the basis for ultrasound diathermy, a common therapeutic use of ultrasound. At the low energy levels used in diagnostic ultrasound, the biologic effect of absorption is negligible, however.

Reflection is the redirection of a portion of the ultrasound beam back toward its source. Reflection gives rise to echoes and forms the basis of diagnostic ultrasound scanning. Whenever the sound beam passes from a tissue of one acoustic impedance to a tissue of a different acoustic impedance, a small portion of the beam will be reflected and the remainder will continue on. We shall take a closer look at this process in a minute.

Scattering occurs when the beam encounters an interface which is irregular and smaller than the sound beam. As the name suggests, the portion of the beam which interacts with this interface is "scattered" in all directions. This is similar to what happens to a cream pie when it is thrown in a face—the cream is splattered in many directions. There is no reason for the clinical ultrasonographer to know much about scattering other than that it occurs. Since the interfaces which produce scattering are small, only a small percentage of the beam is involved. (The portion of the beam which is "scattered" directly backward will return to the transducer and produce an echo—known as a non-specular reflection.)

REFLECTION AND ECHO PRODUCTION

We need to examine the process of ultrasonic reflection and echo production in a little detail since it is the basis of B-mode scanning. Also there seems to be a great deal of confusion and misconception concerning this phenomenon, particularly in regard to "resolution" of ultrasound systems.

Reflection occurs—that is, an echo is produced—whenever the ultrasound beam passes from a tissue of one acoustic impedance to a tissue of a different acoustic impedance. This is also known as crossing an acoustic impedance mismatch or as crossing an acoustic interface. The large number of terms used to describe this probably helps account for the confusion. We will refer to this as an acoustic interface or simply "interface." An **interface** occurs whenever two tissues of differing acoustic impedance are in contact with each other.

Now all we need to know is what is "acoustic impedance"? Elementary, my dear Watson. The **acoustic impedance** of a tissue is the product of the density of the tissue and the speed of sound in the tissue. This is often written as: $Z = p \times c$, where Z = the acoustic impedance, p = the density of the tissue, and c = the speed of sound in the tissue. But the speed of sound in soft tissues is assumed to be a constant (1540 meters per second) so that the only thing which affects the acoustic impedance is the density of the tissue. This simplifies matters greatly. For our purposes we can assume that the acoustic impedance is the same thing as the density of a tissue; therefore, an interface occurs every time tissues of different density are in contact with each other. It takes only very small density differences to make an interface: water, blood cells, fat, liver cells, bile, bile duct walls, blood vessel walls, and connective or fibrous tissue all have sufficiently differing densities to create interfaces. This is one of the reasons ultrasound has proved so useful in abdominal and pelvic examinations: there is a tremendous amount of information about the soft tissues in the ultrasound beam. (The X-ray beam, by contrast, cannot differentiate these small differences in density; water, blood cells, liver cells, bile, bile ducts, blood vessels, and connective and fibrous tissue all appear gray to the X-ray. Even though CT body scanners have excellent resolution, the picture quality is limited by the very small density differences, too small to be detected by X-ray.)

When the sound beam crosses an interface, only a small percentage of it is reflected. The remainder continues on through the tissues where it can be reflected by other interfaces. The amount of sound which is reflected at an interface determines how much amplitude the returning echo will have or how "loud" the echo will be. This amount depends on how great the difference is between the two acoustic impedances which make up the interface. If the difference is very small, only a small percentage of the sound will be reflected; if the difference is large, a large portion will be reflected.

It would seem logical that large echoes would be desirable, but actually this is not the case. Ideally only enough of the beam should be reflected to enable the echo to be detected by the scanner; we want the rest of the beam to be available for creating other echoes. If too large a portion of the beam is reflected at an interface (producing a very loud echo), there is too little of the sound left to produce echoes from other interfaces deeper in the tissue. This is why ultrasound scanners cannot "see" through bowel gas or bone. The difference in acoustic impedance between soft tissue and gas or bone is very large, so large in fact that most of the beam is reflected and none is left to continue deeper. For example, at a soft tissue–bone interface about 70 per cent of the beam is reflected. It takes only two interfaces like this to exhaust the sound. For a soft tissue–gas interface the percentage is over 99 per cent. We can see that bone and gas are the ultrasonic equivalent of a stone wall; nothing gets through them. We should also notice that we are talking about percentage reflection. No matter how powerful the ultrasound beam, the same percentage will be reflected. If we use a louder beam we will get a louder echo but we won't penetrate the gas or bone. It's the same situation as shining a light at a mirror—no matter how bright the light you cannot see through the mirror: you just get a lot of glare. This is important because many people seem to believe that they can blast the sound beam through bowel gas by turning up the power. Although turning up the power makes more echoes, these echoes are mostly artifacts and have no relation to the underlying tissue. Because the problem of artifacts is so great we shall discuss it in greater detail in Chapter 5.

(*Extra reading for aggressive students department:* Why are the acoustic impedances of soft tissue and gas or bone so different? You'll remember that acoustic impedance, Z, is actually the product of density and speed of sound. For soft tissues the speed of sound is nearly constant so only the density factor is involved in changing the value of Z. However, the speed of sound in gas is much slower than in soft tissue and in bone it is much higher. Gas is also much less dense than soft tissue and bone is much more dense. Therefore there are large changes in both the density *and* the speed of sound so the difference in Z is huge.)

There is another term, **refraction,** which is sometimes confused with reflection. Refraction describes what happens to the beam which is not reflected but continues on through the interface. The direction of this beam is changed very slightly and this slight direction change is referred to as refraction. In soft tissues this change is so small that it is of no practical importance to the clinical ultrasonographer. (Refraction is important when the beam crosses a soft tissue–bone interface: another reason why the good ultrasonographer will not scan across this type of interface.)

Specular and Non-specular Reflections

Interfaces give rise to two types of reflections, specular and non-specular.

Specular reflections occur when the interface is larger than the sound beam. Specular reflections have the property that the angle of the reflection is equal to the angle of incidence. We are all familiar with a common type of specular reflection: a pool ball on a pool table. If we shoot the ball against one of the cushions, it will bounce off at the same angle at which we shot it (assuming, of course, we are not doing anything fancy like putting spin on the ball). If we shoot it head on into the cushion, it will come directly back at us; if we shoot it at an angle it will not come back to us.

Figure 1–3 illustrates specular reflections as they pertain to ultrasound.

It is obvious that unless the ultrasound beam strikes a specular reflector nearly head on, the echo will not come back to the transducer but will go angling off into the tissue. The scientific expression for this is that the echo has an "angle dependence." This simply means that the strength of the echo depends not only on the differences in acoustic impedance at the interface, but

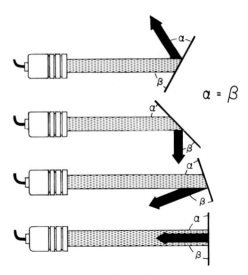

$\alpha = \beta$

Figure 1–3. Specular reflections occur when the reflecting interface is larger than the sound beam. The angle at which the echo is reflected is equal to the angle at which the pulse hit the reflector. The echo will return to the transducer *only if* this is a right angle or very close to it.

also on the angle at which the beam strikes the interface.

Specular echoes are very common in abdominal scanning. The capsule of the liver and kidney, the aorta and major vessels, the gallbladder, and the bile ducts are all examples of specular reflectors. Almost all the echoes in bi-stable scans are specular. This is why the technique of bi-stable scanning involves compound scanning. The transducer must be continually angled and moved so that the sound beam has a chance to strike the reflectors at many different angles, eventually finding an angle which will allow the echo to return to the transducer. Bi-stable scanning is discussed in Chapter 12.

Specular echoes are something of a problem in gray-scale ultrasound. One of the goals of gray-scale scanning is the preservation of echo amplitude information. Each shade of gray corresponds to a certain range of echo amplitude and might be expected to be the same every time this type of echo is received. But since the amplitude of a specular echo depends not only upon the nature of the interface but on the angle as well, it is clear that the shade of gray will vary widely, depending upon where the transducer is positioned when the echo is received. Thus, the echoes from the capsule of the kidney may be stronger, the same as, or weaker than the echoes from the renal parenchyma, depending upon the beam angle. There is no way to avoid this problem; however, it is not too difficult to live with as long as we recognize that the shade of gray of a specular echo does not have much significance.

Non-specular reflections occur when the interface is smaller than the sound beam. As we shall see, the sound beam from a modern, well-focused transducer is on the order of 10 millimeters in diameter. Therefore, interfaces smaller than 10 millimeters will give rise to non-specular reflections. Many small parenchymal tissue echoes fall into this category, such as those arising between cells and small vessels, hepatic cells and fat cells, and renal cells and renal tubules. In contrast to specular echoes, the amplitude of a non-specular echo is independent of the beam angle. That this should be so is obvious if we consider that the small non-specular interface is always surrounded by the beam and hence there really is no such thing as an incident angle as far as the interface is concerned. Although not dependent on the angle of incidence, the amplitude of non-specular echoes is usually much less than the amplitude of specular echoes—usually by at least 30 dB—because the interfaces are so much smaller and consequently cannot reflect as much of the beam as the larger, specular interfaces.

Non-specular echoes are not used much in bi-stable scanning, although they can be detected as readily with bi-stable equipment as with gray-scale. The problem is that, because these reflections are so weak, the scan must be performed at a high sensitivity or gain level and so many echoes are received that the picture becomes totally white (sensitivity and gain will be discussed in Chapter 3).

Gray-scale scanning, however, makes good use of these reflections. Because the differing amplitudes of many echoes are recorded in different shades of gray, it is possible to scan at the high-gain settings required to receive non-specular echoes and still maintain a useful image. The picture is full of echoes but instead of being all white, as it would be on a bi-stable scan, it is composed of many shades of gray. Non-specular reflections are also well suited to gray-scale scanners, since the echo amplitude is independent of beam angle; the shade of gray (corresponding to the amplitude) of an echo is more nearly constant and more diagnostically useful.

RESOLUTION

The problem of resolution in ultrasound is similar to the weather: everybody talks about it but nobody does anything about it. Improved resolution is a goal as laudable as motherhood or apple pie. After all, if the ultrasound picture could show smaller interfaces it just stands to reason that the pictures would look better and be more diagnostically useful. Therefore, most equipment manufacturers and many authors like to stress the importance of improving resolution. Now we do not wish to be on the opposite side of any popular movement, be it motherhood or improving resolution in ultrasound systems, but we do think that this concept has received more than its fair share of attention. It is undoubtedly true that improving the resolution of an imaging system will improve the picture quality. But it is not as certain that this will result in improved diagnosis. The diagnostic value of an ultrasound scan is dependent upon many factors, and resolution is only one of them. Scanning technique, number and type of artifacts, scan reproducibility, quality of the hard copy system, and body habitus of the patient are some of the other factors which are at least as important as resolution in determining the overall diagnostic utility of a scan. While it is important to have an idea of what limits resolution and how to improve it, it is just as important to improve all the aspects of the scanning process.

The reason that no one does anything about resolution is simply that there is not much more that can be done. Modern scanners are capable of resolution that is near the limits imposed by the physical considerations of the pulse echo process. Let us briefly examine these limitations.

Resolution is the ability to separate two closely spaced interfaces. Resolution is usually expressed as a distance, 3 millimeters, for example. If the ultrasound system has a resolution capability of 3 millimeters, it means that two small interfaces

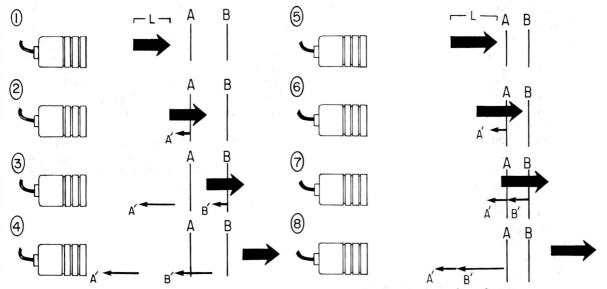

Figure 1–4. Diagrammatic representation of the effect of pulse length on axial resolution.
  Lines 1 to 4 show the situation where two interfaces, A and B, are separated by more than one-half the pulse length, L. The echoes from A and B (A' and B') do not overlap and the transducer sees two separate echoes.
  Lines 5 to 8 show the situation when A and B are closer than one-half L. In this case, the echoes A' and B' overlap and the transducer sees only a single echo.

spaced only 3 millimeters apart will appear as two separate echoes in the image. However, if the two interfaces are closer together than this, 2 millimeters, for example, they will appear as a single echo in the picture. (*Comparative terminology department:* In evaluating radiologic systems, resolution is usually expressed in terms of line pairs per distance rather than simple distance; in this case the larger the number of line pairs, the greater the resolution.)

Ultrasonic resolution has two components: axial and lateral. **Axial resolution** refers to resolution along the path of the sound beam. Axial resolution is dependent upon many factors, including the type and quality of the electronics in the scanner and the transducer design and construction, but the ultimate limitation is the physical constraints of the ultrasound beam itself.

We have been speaking of the ultrasound "beam," but actually we mean a series of ultrasound pulses. Each pulse has a small, but definite, length. This is easily found by multiplying the speed of sound by the duration of the pulse. For a typical gray-scale scanner, each pulse lasts about 1 microsecond. (A microsecond is one-millionth of a second and is abbreviated, μsecond.) 1 μsecond × 1540 meters per second = 1.54 millimeters as the length of the pulse.

Physical principles state that the resolution can be no better than ½ the pulse length, so the axial resolution of a system with a 1 μsecond pulse can be no better than 1.54/2 = 0.77 millimeter. Figure 1–4 illustrates why resolution can be no better than ½ of the pulse length.

Physical principles also state that the axial resolution can be no better than one wavelength. The wavelengths of commonly used ultrasound frequencies are:

1.6 MHz = 0.96 millimeter
2.25 MHz = 0.68 millimeter
3.5 MHz = 0.44 millimeter
5.0 MHz = 0.31 millimeter

We can see that as frequency increases, resolution also increases. However, it is important to notice that overall resolution is limited not only by the frequency but also by the pulse length (pulse length is dependent upon transducer characteristics). In actual practice, neither of these factors is as important as the limited resolution of the oscilloscope or TV monitor which is used to display the picture. The point to remember in all this is that frequency is only one of many factors affecting resolution, and simply using a higher frequency transducer does not guarantee that resolution will be improved.

Lateral resolution refers to resolution perpendicular to the axis of the sound beam. This can also be thought of as side-to-side resolution. Lateral resolution is dependent upon the size or diameter of the ultrasound beam; the smaller the beam the better the resolution. Figure 1–5 illustrates that lateral resolution is limited to the beam width. If two interfaces are closer together than the beam width, then they will both give rise to an echo at the same time and only a single echo will be received by the transducer.

Beam width is a very complicated and poorly defined area of ultrasound. Most beams do not start and stop abruptly but instead taper off. At what point do we say that the beam "ends"? Depending on what point is chosen, the same beam can appear very narrow or very wide. Therefore, statements as to beam widths must be taken with several large grains of salt, much as claims about the wattage of stereo equipment. Still, depending upon how they are focused, some transducers function as if they had very narrow beams and others as if they had broad beams. (We will look into transducers in more detail in Chapter 2.) In the early 1970's a standard transducer performed as if it had a beam width of 2 centi-

meters, and this has been the basis for the frequent statement that ultrasound scanning cannot resolve lesions less than 2 to 3 centimeters in size. However, transducer technology has come a long way in the last few years and there are now several transducers on the market which perform as if they had beam widths on the order of 1 centimeter.

We can see that lateral resolution is not as good as axial resolution. Although the large differences which were present a few years ago have decreased, the overall resolution of any B-mode scanning system will still be limited by the lateral resolution of the transducer used and, under most circumstances, will be between 1 and 2 centimeters. (In certain situations the resolution may be improved to 5 millimeters.)

BIOLOGIC EFFECTS

High intensity ultrasound waves can permanently alter the structure of the tissue through which they pass. These effects range from slight warming of the tissue to total necrosis and destruction. The power levels which produce these changes are many orders of magnitude greater than the power levels used for diagnostic B-scanning, however. The power output or intensity of the ultrasound beam is measured in watts per square centimeter (W/cm^2) when biologic effects are being considered. There has been extensive research on the safety of ultrasound in recent years and no adverse effects have ever been demonstrated at intensities less than 100 milliwatts per square centimeter (a milliwatt is one-thousandth of a watt). The peak intensity, that is, the intensity at the height of the pulse, for present ultrasound B-scanners is less than 100 watts per square centimeter. Since the pulse is actually on about one one-thousandth of the time (the remainder of the time the scanner is "listening for the echo"), the temporal average intensity is only a thousandth of the peak intensity or less than 100 milliwatts per square centimeter. Actually the latest generation of gray-scale scanners have temporal average power outputs of about 20 milliwatts per square centimeter.

The American Institute of Ultrasound in Medicine established a Committee on Bio-

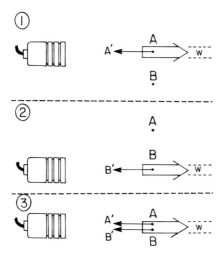

Figure 1–5. Lateral resolution is limited to beam width. If interfaces *A* and *B* are separated by more than the beam width, *W*, then, as the transducer is moved across them, two separate echoes *A'* and *B'* will be generated (Lines 1 and 2). However, if *A* and *B* are closer together than the beam width, the echoes *A'* and *B'* will arrive at the transducer simultaneously and be recorded as a single echo (Line 3).

logic Effects to study the problem of possible toxic effects of ultrasound scanning. In August, 1975, this committee issued the following statement, which summarizes the knowledge of the biologic effects of diagnostic level ultrasound:

Statement on Mammalian in Vivo Ultrasonic Biological Effects

In the low megahertz frequency range there have been (as of this date) no demonstrated significant biological effects in mammalian tissues exposed to intensities* below 100 mW/cm. Furthermore, for ultrasonic exposure times** less than 500 seconds and greater than one second, such effects have not been demonstrated even at higher intensities, when the product of intensity* and exposure time** is less than 50 joules/cm.

---

*Spatial peak, temporal average as measured in a free field in water.
**Total time; this includes off-time as well as on-time for a repeated-pulse regime.

All of the commercially available ultrasound scanners have power outputs well within this safety range.

PERSPECTIVE

It is time to stop and count heads; we have made it through the worst of the physics and we hope that no one got lost along the way. From now on the discussions will be more practical in orientation but we will often refer to the physical principles we have just been over. At the risk of beating a dead horse, we want to reiterate that it is impossible to be a good ultrasonographer unless you have some understanding of where the echoes come from and why; only then can the more subtle problems, such as artifacts, be comprehended and dealt with; only then can the ultrasound literature be read with enough understanding to separate valuable articles from the potboilers; and only then can scanning techniques be modified and improved.

Chapter 2

TRANSDUCERS

The transducer has been described as the "heart" of the ultrasound system. While this may not be the best possible metaphor (we prefer "ear"), it does point up the importance of the transducer in the ultrasonic imaging process. Most ultrasound facilities have only one ultrasound machine and the ultrasonographer can do little to change its physical capacities. By contrast, transducers come in a bewildering number of sizes, shapes, and frequencies, and because of their relatively modest cost each ultrasound facility usually will have more than one. New types are being developed with the regularity of Detroit car models and each new journal or salesman's visit is likely to suggest the need for acquiring a new model.

What is the difference between various types of transducers and what, if any, effect will changing transducers have on the ultrasound image? Is it necessary or even desirable to own more than one transducer? If you do own more than one, when should each be used? Is there a good theoretic basis for preferring one model over another or should the ultrasonographer try all of them out on each patient? Under what circumstances will resolution be improved if a higher frequency transducer is used? When will resolution be improved by using a lower frequency transducer?

Most of these questions do not have definite answers; if they did, then we could just list them and this chapter would be unnecessary. Unfortunately, life is not so simple. The only question we can answer without equivocation is that regarding the desirability of using more than one transducer, and the answer is a definite "yes." The remainder of the questions must be answered by the individual ultrasonographer at the time the scan is being performed. To do this he or she must have some basic understanding of how transducers work and what to expect from the different styles and models.

THE PIEZOELECTRIC EFFECT

The term "piezo" is derived from a Greek word meaning pressure, so piezoelectric translates into pressure-electric. This refers to a property of certain crystals which causes them to emit electricity when pressed or deformed. Conversely, when electricity is applied to a piezoelectric crystal it changes the shape of the crystal.

This phenomenon has many uses besides ultrasound. One with which many of us are familiar is the phonograph. When amplified record players first became available, a piezoelectric crystal was attached to the needle and this crystal generated the small electric currents which were then amplified and played over a loudspeaker. Crystal phonograph cartridges remained popular until the late 1960's and, if you have a vintage hi-fi system, it is quite possible that it utilizes a piezoelectric crystal for a pick-up. (For the most part, crystals have been supplanted by magnetic cartridges in present-day stereo systems.)

Figure 2–1 illustrates the piezoelectric effect as it is utilized in an ultrasound transducer. When a high voltage, between 300 and 700 volts, is applied to opposite faces of the crystal, it expands slightly. If the voltage is turned off the crystal returns to its original size. If the voltage were reapplied, but with opposite polarity (that is, if the positive and negative electrodes were switched), the crystal would shrink slightly. These tiny expansions and contractions of the crystal generate the small pressure waves which are transmitted as the ultrasound pulse. When the crystal is placed in contact with the patient's skin

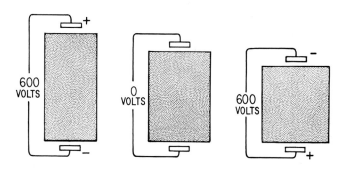

Figure 2–1. When a voltage is applied to a piezoelectric crystal, it either expands or contracts, depending upon the polarity of the voltage. Conversely, if the crystal is physically compressed or stretched, it will generate a voltage in the electrodes.

these expansions and contractions cause pressure waves in the tissue and create the ultrasound beam. When an echo returns to the crystal the small pressure waves deform it slightly, causing a tiny voltage to appear in the electrodes. The greater the amplitude of the echo, the more the crystal is deformed and the higher the voltage generated. (This voltage is in the range of 1 to 1000 millivolts [1000 millivolts = 1 volt], quite small when compared to the large voltage used to initiate the pulse.)

(Short quiz: If the echoes received from a typical abdominal scan generate voltages ranging from 1 to 1000 millivolts, what range of echo amplitude does this represent in decibels?

Answer: Recall the definition of the decibel: $dB = 20 \log \dfrac{E_2}{E_1}$. A factor of 10 is equivalent to 20 decibels. To go from 1 millivolt to 1000 millivolts requires three factors of 10: $10 \times 10 \times 10 = 1000$, so this is equivalent to 60 decibels.
This could also be calculated directly as:

$$20 \log \frac{1000}{1} = 20 \times 3 = 60 \text{ dB}.)$$

There are several types of crystals which possess piezoelectric properties. Quartz is an example of a naturally occurring piezoelectric crystal, but many synthetic materials also have piezoelectric qualities and have several advantages over quartz. At present virtually all transducers for medical ultrasound purposes are made of lead titanate zirconate, although the exact recipes for various models differ, and many of the details of their construction are industrial secrets.
There is one practical matter to keep in mind when dealing with synthetic crystals:

the effect of heat. Synthetic piezoelectric crystals are constructed by crystallizing a ceramic material in the presence of a strong electric field. This "polarizes" the crystal and makes it piezoelectric. If the crystal is reheated in the absence of an electric field it can lose its polarization. For this reason, transducers should never be heat-sterilized.

FREQUENCY

The frequency of a transducer is determined by how many times the crystal expands and contracts per second. There are two ways of controlling this.
The first simply involves cycling the voltage applied to the crystal at whatever frequency is desired. If we wanted a 1.6 MHz transducer, we would cycle the voltage 1.6 million times per second; if we wanted 2.25 MHz, we would cycle at 2.25 MHz. (Although this may sound difficult, it is actually quite simple for the electronics circuit designer.) There are some advantages to controlling frequency this way. To begin, we know exactly what the frequency is. Also, if we wanted to change frequency, we could simply turn a dial and change the excitation rate without having to touch or change the transducer. Some Doppler systems use this type of excitation of the crystal.
There is a major problem with using this method in pulse-echo systems, however, and that is pulse length. As we saw in Chapter 1, the resolution of the ultrasound system is limited by the pulse length; to get high resolution we must have a very short pulse, ideally only a single cycle. This is not possible if an oscillating voltage is used to drive the crystal at a fixed frequency. Fortunately, there is a method

of controlling crystal frequency while maintaining short pulse lengths; and this makes use of the property known as resonance.

Resonance is defined as a reinforcement of sound by sympathetic vibration. This definition probably seems a bit obscure, and it is easiest to understand resonance by considering some everyday examples.

We are all familiar with musical glasses. After an elegant meal someone lines up all the partially empty wine glasses and starts banging on them with a knife. The glasses "ring" when struck, producing a tone with a definite pitch. However, each glass produces a different tone, depending on how much wine it contains — the more wine, the higher the pitch. If the dinner guest is musically inclined, he can often play a tune on the glasses. How is it that identical wine glasses can produce different notes when struck by the same knife? Resonance, of course. When the glass is struck it starts to vibrate and the vibrations produce pressure waves in the air, which we hear as sound. The pitch of the sound depends on the frequency at which the glass is vibrating. The amount of wine in the glass determines the frequency of the vibrations and hence the pitch of the note.

A xylophone works on exactly the same principle. The wooden bar of the xylophone is struck with a stick and starts to vibrate. The vibrations produce pressure waves in the air which we hear as sound. The pitch of the sound is determined by the frequency at which the bar vibrates and this frequency is determined by the size of the bar.

Immediately after being struck the bar starts to vibrate. Now the edge of the bar and air make an interface at which sound will be reflected (just as tissues of different densities make an interface), and when the sound wave (vibration) reaches this interface a portion of it will be reflected back into the bar. The sound wave then travels back through the bar until it reaches the opposite edge where it encounters another bar-air interface. A portion of the wave is again reflected back through the bar. This process continues, with the sound wave bouncing back and forth between the two edges of the bar until it finally dies out by attenuation.

Let us now consider the effect of wavelength (and therefore frequency) on this rebounding sound wave. First we will consider a wavelength which is not related to the size of the bar. Figure 2–2 shows what happens as this wave moves back and forth. The amplitude at any point within the bar is nearly zero, because after a very few cycles the wave is all jumbled up on top of itself. Since the amplitude at any point is actually the sum of all the waves that are present at that point, the jumbled up waves tend to cancel each other out and the net result is nearly zero. This wave is said to be **out of phase** and will die out instantly because of self-attenuation.

Figure 2–3 shows the situation when the wavelength is twice as long as the size of the bar (or we can think of this as the size

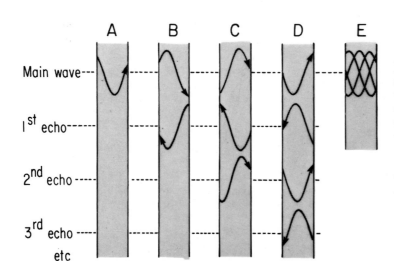

Figure 2–2. When the wavelength is not related to the size of the vibrating object, the effective amplitude may be nearly zero. *A* to *D* show the main wave and some of the echo waves generated as internal reflections, or resonance, occur. In this diagram we have shown each wave on a separate line for simplicity. Actually, all the waves are superimposed, as in *E*, and tend to cancel each other out.

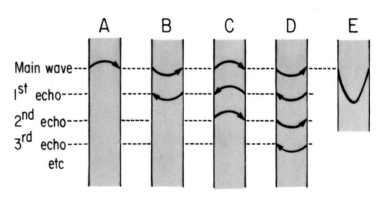

Figure 2–3. When the size of the vibrating object is one-half a wavelength the effective amplitude of the wave is increased. A to D show the main wave and some of the echo waves generated by internal reflections, or resonance. In *D*, we have shown each wave on a separate line for simplicity. Actually, all the waves are superimposed, as in *E*. The resulting amplitude is the sum of all the waves and is increased.

of the bar being one half a wavelength). We can see that the wave will always be reflected as it crosses zero amplitude and that the reflected waves, instead of being all jumbled up, will superimpose on each other. Instead of canceling each other out, the reflected waves will actually reinforce each other and the amplitude will be increased. This wave is said to be **in phase.** An in phase wave will be continually reinforced while an out of phase wave will be extinguished. The size of the bar determines which wavelength will be in phase and consequently at which frequency the bar will vibrate.

(*Advanced study department:* What would happen to a wave if the size of the bar were one and one half times the wavelength? Would the wave be in or out of phase? *Answer:* If we were to construct drawings similar to Figures 2–2 and 2–3 for these situations, we would see that as long as the size of the bar is equal to an *odd* number of ½ wavelengths the wave will be in phase. If the size of the bar equals an *even* number of ½ wavelengths the wave will be totally out of phase. The various odd number of ½ wavelengths which are in phase with the bar are known as the **harmonics** of the bar.)

This whole process of internal, back-and-forth reflection of sound waves is **resonance.** Because of resonance some frequencies (the resonant frequencies) will be enhanced and others will be suppressed. Knowing about harmonics or resonant frequencies is not so important; the thing to understand is that the frequency at which an object vibrates, be it a xylophone bar, a wine glass, a guitar string, or a piezoelectric crystal, depends upon its size. If a xylophone bar is made shorter, or a guitar

string shortened by placing a finger across it, the bar and the string will vibrate at a higher frequency (corresponding to the shorter wavelength which will then be in phase).

The same situation holds for the transducer crystal. The frequency is determined by the thickness of the crystal. In pulse-echo ultrasound the crystal is "shocked" by a single, extremely short pulse of electricity (analogous to striking a xylophone bar with a stick) and then "resonates" at a frequency determined by its thickness.

BANDWIDTH

Under ideal circumstances a transducer would emit only a single frequency, determined by its crystal thickness. In practice, however, this is not possible. Slight imperfections in the crystal, non-parallel faces, irregularities in the face, coupling of waves into the load and backing material, length of exciting pulse, and many other factors all combine to broaden the frequency of the transducer. (Sometimes these factors are deliberately manipulated so that the transducer will have a large frequency spectrum.) Even though a transducer is designed to operate at a single frequency it actually emits ultrasound waves of many frequencies on either side of the main frequency. The range of frequencies produced is known as the bandwidth of the transducer. A transducer with a large bandwidth emits a wide range of frequencies while one with a narrow bandwidth sends out only a few frequencies. There have been considerable technical advances in transducer construction in recent years and modern transducers can have quite narrow bandwidths. Figure 2–4 shows an actual

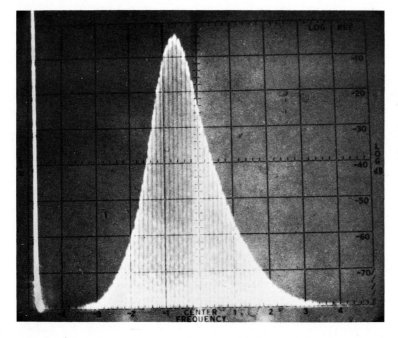

Figure 2–4. The frequency spectrum of a modern transducer can be quite narrow. This is the actual spectrum of a transducer with a nominal "frequency" of 2.25 MHz. The largest portion of the output is between 1.5 and 3.0 MHz. The peak frequency is 2.15 MHz and each horizontal scale division is equal to 0.5 MHz. (Courtesy of Aerotech Laboratories.)

spectral analysis of a current ultrasound transducer. Most of the frequencies produced are closely centered about the peak frequency of 2.15 MHz. There is no significant output at frequencies of 1.0 and 3.5 MHz.

The practical importance of this is that although we speak of transducers as if they emitted only a single frequency (and hence a specific resolution and single attenuation coefficient), we are really dealing with a band of frequencies. The actual transducer has a range of resolution and attenuation coefficients; and if these ranges are large (that is, if the bandwidth is wide), there may be so much overlap between transducers that they behave in the same manner. Therefore, if your transducers don't have narrow bandwidths, you may not be able to discern any difference between them in use. Figure 2–5 illustrates this situation.

EFFECTS OF FREQUENCY

Assuming that we have narrow bandwidth transducers of differing frequencies available, is there some theoretic reason to use more than one frequency when scanning? Obviously, the answer is "yes" (we told you that earlier). Let us briefly summarize the advantages of the differing frequencies.

We saw in Chapter 1 that the axial resolution improves as frequency is increased. Lateral resolution also improves because higher frequency transducers can be more precisely focused than lower frequency transducers. (Actually most of the perceptible improvement in resolution is due to the improvement of lateral resolution since axial resolution in practice is limited by factors other than frequency, such as pulse length and monitor resolution.)

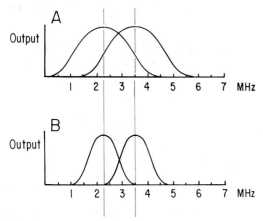

Figure 2–5. If transducers do not have narrow bandwidths, there may be little difference in the pictures they produce. In *A*, the bandwidths of a 2.5 and 3.5 MHz transducer overlap significantly because they are so wide. There is little difference in the actual sound beam. In *B*, however, the bandwidths are narrow and these 2.5 and 3.5 MHz transducers have very different outputs.

Attenuation is greater for higher frequencies, however, and this limits the situations in which they can be used, particularly in abdominal and pelvic B-scanning. It does no good to have a high resolution beam if the attenuation is so great that it cannot reach its target. A 5 MHz transducer may have better resolution than a 2.25 MHz transducer, but the attenuation of the 5 MHz beam is more than twice as great and it has, therefore, less than half the useful working range of the 2.25 MHz beam. In clinical scanning a 5 MHz transducer gives excellent images up to a depth of 3 or 4 centimeters but is worthless for deeper structures. Lower frequency transducers give better pictures of deep structures than the higher frequency models. Although the resolution of a 1.6 MHz transducer is inferior to that of a 2.25 MHz one, in many situations, such as in the case of a large patient or in tissue with high attenuation such as cirrhotic liver, the picture quality will be better if the 1.6 MHz transducer is used.

PULSE LENGTH

When the piezoelectric crystal is "shocked" by the electric voltage, it "rings," much like a gong which has been struck with a mallet. Under normal circumstances the ringing might go on for several microseconds before it died out. This would be unacceptable for pulse-echo purposes, as it would generate a very long pulse, and, as we have seen in Chapter 1, a long pulse means poor resolution. Under ideal circumstances we would like the crystal to ring for only a single cycle. To stop a gong from ringing all we have to do is touch it or apply a wad of cotton to it; this is known as "damping" the gong. (Those who are pianists will be familiar with the "damper pedal," which controls the damping of the piano strings: when the pedal is depressed the strings ring for a long time; when it is released, damping is applied and the sound stops.)

Damping is also applied to transducer crystals to limit the pulse length. This is accomplished by placing an acoustically absorbent material in contact with the back face of the crystal; this material absorbs the vibrational energy and limits the ringing. The composition and thickness of the damping material must be carefully chosen and matched to the type and frequency of the crystal if the damping is to be effective. The damping material also prevents the ultrasound wave from being transferred to the transducer case. If the wave were propagated in the case it would give rise to all sorts of internal reverberations as it echoed around and this would be picked up by the crystal as spurious echoes (it might also make the ultrasonographer's fingers tingle). A well-damped transducer emits a short pulse in the forward direction only.

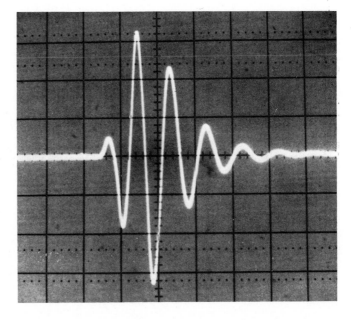

Figure 2–6. The pulse of a well-damped transducer is limited to less than 2 microseconds. This is a photograph of an actual transducer pulse. It is nearly totally damped in 1.5 microseconds, and yields a pulse length of slightly over 2 millimeters. Each horizontal division equals 0.5 microsecond. (Courtesy of Aerotech Laboratories.)

Figure 2–6 shows the pulse from a well-damped transducer shocked for 0.5 microsecond; it consists of only three cycles with significant amplitude and has a duration of about one and a half microseconds which corresponds to a pulse length of slightly over 2 millimeters.

NON-FOCUSED TRANSDUCERS

If the face of the transducer crystal is placed directly in contact with the patient, the transducer is said to be non-focused. (Some non-focused transducers may have a thin protective coating over the crystal face, but this coating does not affect the beam pattern or focusing as long as it is thin and uniform.) Figure 2–7 illustrates the beam pattern from a non-focused transducer. There are two areas of interest. The first is known as the Fresnel zone and is the area close to the transducer face (also known as the "near field"). Within the Fresnel zone the beam diameter is relatively constant and approximately equal to the diameter of the transducer crystal. The beam is uneven in this zone, however; that is, the amplitude of the beam varies widely at different points in the zone. The differences can be quite large, on the order of 10 to 20 decibels or even more. This does not present a great problem in bi-stable scanning where the amplitude of individual echoes is not important, but it is a definite disadvantage in the use of gray scale where echo amplitude information is desired. The uniformity of the beam can be improved somewhat by special electrode designs and focal damping of the crystal, but it cannot be completely eliminated.

Following the Fresnel zone, in the far field, is the Fraunhofer zone. The beam is uniform in the Fraunhofer zone. However, it diverges rapidly and, because of this, there is increased attenuation and loss of lateral resolution.

The depth of the Fresnel zone is directly related to the size of the transducer face and inversely related to the wavelength of the ultrasound. The Fresnel zone can, therefore, be lengthened by using a transducer with a larger face or lower frequency or both.

Non-focused transducers are adequate for many ultrasound applications — most echoencephalography and bi-stable abdominal scanning, for example. However, for gray-scale abdominal scanning it is necessary to use a focused transducer for best resolution and echo amplitude sensitivity.

FOCUSED TRANSDUCERS

As is the case with visible light, ultrasound waves can be focused by use of lenses. The actual physics of this process is quite complicated and much of it poorly understood. While this may be a problem for the transducer designer, as ultrasonographers all we need to know is that improvements in transducer focusing are constantly being made and that present transducers manage to produce a quite narrow beam of fairly uniform amplitude over a long working range. Figure 2–8 shows a beam profile of a well-focused transducer. There are only a few important concepts to keep in mind regarding focused transducers.

Most present-day transducers are "internally focused." This means that the crystal and lens are inside the transducer case and that the face of the transducer is flat. The advantage of such transducers is that good skin contact can be maintained and defocusing and attenuation due to poor acoustic coupling at the transducer-skin interface are minimized. "Externally focused" transducers have a concave face which makes it difficult to maintain good transducer-skin contact. Figure 2–9 shows a diagrammatic cross-section of a transducer.

Several terms are used to describe the

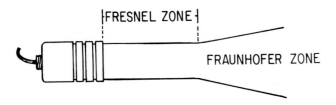

FRESNEL ZONE

FRAUNHOFER ZONE

Figure 2–7. The ultrasonic field of a non-focused transducer has two components. In the near field, or Fresnel zone, the beam width is constant but the intensity fluctuates. In the far field, or Fraunhofer zone, the intensity is constant but the beam diverges rapidly.

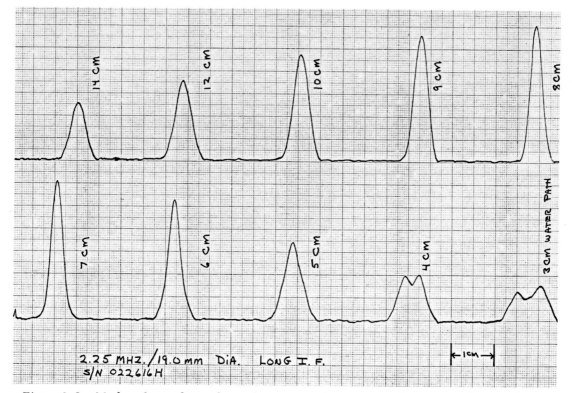

Figure 2-8. Modern focused transducers have narrow beams over a long range. This is a plot of an actual transducer beam. The width is plotted on the horizontal axis while the amplitude is shown on the vertical axis. The distance from the transducer face at which the measurement was taken is written beside each plot. Notice that the plot was made from *right to left* and from *bottom to top.* At 3, 4, and 5 centimeters the beam is rather wide and of low amplitude. From 6 to 12 centimeters the beam is narrow and of good amplitude. (Courtesy of Aerotech Laboratories.)

Figure 2-9. A transducer is complex. This cutaway view of an internally focused transducer shows its components. (Courtesy of Aerotech Laboratories.)

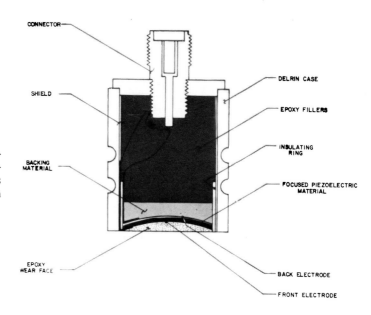

MEDICAL B-SCAN TRANSDUCER

type of focus. "Short," "medium," and "long" are common, as are numbers, such as "6 centimeters" or "10 centimeters." These terms mean different things to different manufacturers; sometimes they refer to the radius of the lens, sometimes the focal point, and sometimes the range of the focal zone. A little intuition is all that is needed here. Obviously a "short" focus will be better suited to working at close range, while "medium" will be useful at depths of 4 to 8 centimeters. "Long" should be utilized when there are deep echoes.

The higher the frequency of the transducer, the better it can be focused. A higher-frequency transducer will usually have a narrower beam width than a transducer of the same diameter but lower frequency.

For transducers of the same frequency, the degree of focusing is directly related to the size of the transducer face; the larger the face, the better the focus. This is why the large, 19 millimeter transducer is more popular for gray-scale B-scanning than the smaller, 13 millimeter transducer. In general it is best to use the largest transducer which can be kept in good skin contact.

Before we leave the topic of beam focusing we should examine what is meant by the expression "beam width." Although we use it frequently and probably have a good intuitive notion of what it means, it is not so easy to make a precise definition. The ultrasound beam is similar to a paint sprayer; there is no sharp edge. Although the sprayer will deposit most of the paint in a small circle, there will be some paint sprayed over a wider area. What constitutes the "size" of the paint spray? Is it where 30 per cent of the paint is sprayed? 50 per cent? 90 per cent? Clearly we must pick some arbitrary amount—say 50 per cent—and define the "size" of the spray as that area in which 50 per cent of the paint falls.

A similar arbitrary definition of ultrasound beam width must be selected. Instead of using the amount of sound (which is what we did with the paint) we use the amplitude of the sound beam. Thus we say the beam "ends" when the amplitude decreases by 3 dB; or 6 dB; or 100 dB. The width of the beam will vary depending on which level is chosen, as illustrated in Figure 2–10.

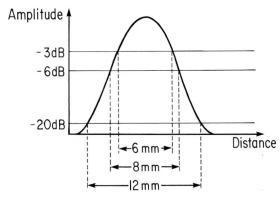

Figure 2–10. "Beam width" varies with the decibel level used to define it. In this example we are examining a single beam profile. The amplitude of the beam is plotted on the vertical axis versus distance on the horizontal axis. If we define the beam "width" as 3dB (this means the beam "ends" when it has decreased 3dB in amplitude), the width is 6 mm. If we call 6dB the end of the beam (this corresponds to a 50 per cent loss of amplitude), the width is 8 mm. At 20dB (a reduction of 90 per cent) the width is 12 mm.

If 3 dB is chosen, the beam will appear to be very narrow since this represents only a 30 per cent reduction from peak amplitude. However, this is not a particularly useful definition for our purposes. Since the echoes we are receiving cover a range of 60 dB, a change of only 3 dB is hardly noticeable. A 20 dB beam width is a more useful definition, and 40 dB is even better. The point to keep in mind is that when the beam widths of two transducers are compared, it is important to know how the beam width is being defined. (As we mentioned in Chapter 1, this same problem occurs in describing the power of stereo equipment; the "watts" of one manufacturer may not be equal to the "watts" of another.)

SPECIAL PURPOSE TRANSDUCERS

Transducers are available in a bewildering variety of sizes, shapes, and frequencies. In addition to those for regular scanning, there are several special purpose models. These include tiny ones which can be attached to needles or probes, rotating models for insertion into bodily orifices, small-face models for fitting between children's ribs, and various grooved and channeled types for guided biopsy. The only type of particular interest to the abdominal and pelvic ultrasonographer are the biopsy transducers. These are essentially the same as a standard transducer with the addition of a central channel in the axis of the sound beam through which a biopsy needle can be passed. The latest models are well focused and produce as good pictures as a standard transducer. There are two types available for B-scanning: one has only a central channel and the other has a notch. The notched models permit the transducer to be removed after the biopsy needle has been positioned. We will discuss the use of these transducers further in Chapter 13.

TRANSDUCERS FOR GENERAL SCANNING

As we said earlier, there are no easy answers as to which transducers to use when, and how many and what type the well-equipped ultrasound lab should have. We have used nearly every available type and frequency and have found situations in which almost every one was uniquely useful. Yet, it is obvious that it is not necessary to own a complete arsenal of transducers to do good work, and we have found that we use only the five shown in Figure 2–11 for almost all of our work.

By far the most useful is a 19 mm diameter, 2.25 MHz, long internal focus model. This is the standard transducer furnished with scanners and the actual specifications may vary slightly from manufacturer to manufacturer. This transducer will handle almost all scanning situations; and, if your laboratory has a limited budget, there is no great need to have any others.

We are somewhat less certain as to which is the next most useful model, but we lean toward a 19 mm diameter, 1.6 MHz, long internal focus. As we shall see in future chapters, despite some loss in resolution, the overall picture quality is often more diagnostically useful with the longer wavelength.

A 5 MHz, short internal focus transducer is helpful for superficial scanning of organs such as the thyroid or testicle or subcutaneous masses. The limited range of this transducer makes it unsuited for general abdominal work except in very small infants. The transducer is available with both 6 mm and 13 mm crystals. In our experience, resolution seems better with the 6 mm crystal, but it is important that the total face diameter of the transducer be at least 10 mm. If the face is smaller than this, it is

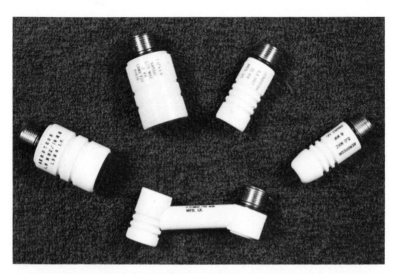

Figure 2–11. A limited number of transducers will suffice for most situations. We use the five shown here. Center: the 3.5 MHz biopsy transducer. Clockwise from left: 1.6 MHz, 19 mm, long internal focus; 2.25 MHz, 19 mm, long internal focus; 3.5 MHz, 13 mm, medium internal focus; 5 MHz, 6 mm, short internal focus with blunt scanning tip.

difficult to scan without distorting the tissue.

We have found that a 13 mm diameter, 3.5 MHz, medium internal focus transducer is often helpful. The resolution of this transducer is better than that of the standard transducer, and the range is only slightly decreased. When dealing with thin patients, excellent pictures can be obtained. The smaller face is useful when it becomes necessary to scan between ribs.

For biopsies we use a 13 mm diameter, 3.5 MHz, medium internal focus transducer with an 18 gauge center channel. This is the same transducer as in the preceding paragraph except that it is adapted for biopsy. We will discuss this transducer further in Chapter 13.

Finally, we will once again stress that the transducer is only one part of the overall imaging process. Picture quality depends not only on the transducer but also on the quality of the ultrasound scanner, the type of electronics and image display, the nature of the patient, and, most importantly, on the skill of the person performing the scan. All the transducers in the world cannot compensate for poor scanning technique.

Chapter 3

SCANNERS

An alternative title for this chapter might have been: "Everything you always wanted to know about an ultrasound scanner, but were afraid to ask" (for fear of having a seizure when someone started talking about RF amplifiers, enveloping, integrated circuits, linear encoders, and the like). Admittedly, electronics is a subject of limited interest to most of us, but we do not have to know anything about electronics to understand how a scanner works, because the concepts are all relatively simple. Manufacturers have been streamlining and simplifying machines; and the modern gray-scale scanners have fewer knobs and are easier to use than the machines of a few years ago; when the images are poor there are only a few adjustments which can be made to improve things. In the next few pages we are going to look inside a "typical" gray-scale scanner to see how the various controls affect the picture and why. Although the external appearance and the optional accessories of the various commercially available scanners are different, they are all very similar electronically and all do pretty much the same thing to the echoes.

It is useful to divide the scanner into three parts: the sounder, the position monitor, and the display system. The sounder consists of the electronic apparatus which generates the pulse, receives the echo, amplifies and processes the resulting electric signal, and feeds it to the display system. The sounder is like a fancy stereo receiver. The position monitor keeps track of the transducer position so that the signals from the sounder can be correctly oriented on the display. (A-mode and M-mode scans do not use a position monitor; the ultrasonographer is expected to know where the transducer is aimed.) The display system produces the image which we view. It may be an oscilloscope, a film, a scan converter, or a combination of these. If we extend the analogy of the sounder and stereo receiver,

the display system is the equivalent of the speakers or headphones.

Does everybody have his tool kit and soldering iron? Good! We are ready to start building a gray-scale scanner from scratch: we shall call our "typical" scanner the "SuperSon-Alpha." Naturally we start with the sounder.

PULSE GENERATOR

The first thing we must do is cause the transducer to send out the pulse. We know that to do this we need to generate a very short electric voltage which will "shock" the crystal and start it ringing. The shorter the shock, the better. One half a microsecond is a good length of time and is about average for most ultrasound machines. There are a lot of electronic doodads available which can generate a short electric voltage: thyratron-controlled capacitor-discharge circuits, silicon control capacitors, blocking oscillators, and the like. You can pick your favorite, we will quickly install it (without worrying about how it works) and proceed to other decisions.

The next matter is how often to repeat the pulse. This will have to represent a compromise. We would like to pulse as rapidly as possible so that we can collect echoes quickly. This will mean that the transducer can be moved over the patient with good speed without leaving skip marks. (As we shall see later on, this is extremely important if real-time scanning is to be done.) On the other hand, the ultrasound pulse travels with a fixed speed (1540 meters/second) and we must allow enough time for the pulse to travel to the interface and return before we start a second pulse; otherwise our pulses and echoes will pile up on top of each other. Now, at 1540 meters per second the pulse will travel 1.54 millimeters per microsecond. Therefore, if we want to be able to receive an echo from a distance of 20 centimeters we will have to allow 260 microsec-onds for the sound pulse to make the jour-ney to the interface and back (total distance traveled is 2×20 cm $= 40$ cm; 40 cm $= 400$ mm; 400 mm $\div 1.54$ mm/μsec $= 260$ μsec), and the maximum pulse rate we could use would be about 3800 pulses per second. For standard B-scanning this is certainly rapid enough to give a continuous picture. Most machines actually use a rate of 1000 pulses per second. This allows plenty of time to receive echoes from deep struc-tures and also allows time for the rest of the sounder to process and amplify the echoes.

There is one final adjustment we must make in our pulse generator and that is voltage. We must select the amount of volt-age with which the transducer crystal is shocked. As we saw in Chapter 2, the greater the voltage, the greater the size change of the transducer and the louder the resulting pulse. Of course, if we use too high a voltage and get a very strong pulse, we may overpower the damping material in the transducer and cause excessive ring-ing of the crystal. This would give an excessively long pulse and decrease the axial resolution (the focusing and lateral resolution would decrease as well). On the other hand, if we use too small a voltage the pulse will be so weak that it will be rapidly attenuated and never reach the in-terfaces. It turns out that between 300 and 600 volts gives a nice pulse, one that has enough amplitude to reach deep interfaces without having an unduly long pulse.

You have probably noticed that we can make further use of this shocking voltage. If we install a control which allows us to vary the voltage over this 300 to 600 volt range we will have a method of controlling the output of the transducer. When a stronger beam is needed to pick up small or distant echoes, we can turn up the volt-age. If the echoes are too loud we can turn it down. Let us install such a control; its of-ficial name is an **attenuator** and it varies the electrical impedance of the circuit to the crystal. (Do not confuse this with acoustic impedance; electrical impedance is similar to electrical resistance and is a concept used only in electric circuit design). Changing the electrical impedance has the effect of changing the voltage applied to the crystal.

The attenuator will also control the size of the electric voltage generated in the crystal by the returning echoes. It will therefore work not only on the transmitted pulse but on the received echoes as well. This makes the attenuator an excellent con-trol for adjusting the overall "gain" or "sen-

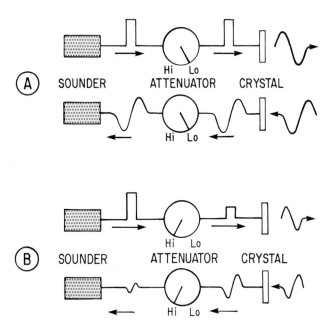

Figure 3–1. The attenuator controls both the output from the transducer and the strength of the electric signal gener-ated by the echo.

A, The attenuator is at low setting. The electric "shocking voltage" from the sounder proceeds through the attenuator to the crystal without any loss in voltage, causing a loud pulse (top line). The elec-tric signal from the returning echo re-turns to the sounder through the attenu-ator without any loss in voltage (bottom line).

B, The attenuator at high setting. The electric "shocking voltage" is attenuated before reaching the crystal and a weaker echo is produced (top line). The electric signal from the echo is also attenuated before it returns to the sounder (bottom line).

sitivity" of the sounder. Figure 3–1 shows the effect of different attenuator settings.

(*Confusing terminology department:* All ultrasound machines have an attenuator but it goes by different names. Some manufacturers call it the "Gain Control," some call it a "Damper Control," some even call it an "Attenuator." Whatever its name, it is the control which is primarily used to set the "gain" on gray-scale scanners. Some scanners have an additional "gain" control which modifies the amplifier. This control is usually set once for the particular transducer being used and is not changed during the course of scanning. We'll discuss this whole confusing business of "gain" and "gain control" in the next section.

Let's just pause a minute for breath. We've finished building the first part of the sounder—the pulse generator. Our "SuperSon-Alpha" uses a shocking voltage of between 300 and 600 volts. This shock is sent to the transducer 1000 times a second so the **pulse rate** is 1000 per second. The shock is very brief, lasting only 0.5 microseconds; this generates an ultrasound pulse which lasts less than 2 microseconds. The electric circuit to the transducer is controlled by an attenuator which changes not only the size of the shocking voltage (and hence the amplitude of the ultrasound pulse) but also the size of the electric voltage generated in the crystal by the returning echo.

Our machine is now sending out pulses and the echoes are returning to the transducer. The crystal in the transducer converts these echoes to very tiny electric voltages. The louder the echo the higher the voltage. The next function of the sounder is to amplify and process these voltages so that they can be sent to the display system.

RADIO FREQUENCY (R.F.) AMPLIFIERS

Before we go further, let's make sure we have an understanding of amplification and "gain." To amplify means to make larger or stronger and an **amplifier** is an electronic device which enlarges and strengthens signals fed into it. We're all familiar with the amplifier in a stereo system which enhances the tiny electric signals from the record and feeds them to the speakers with enough power to break plaster (or leases). When we turn up the "volume" or "loudness" knobs on the stereo we are increasing the amplification of the signal.

The term "gain" is frequently used in ultrasound to refer to the degree of amplification. If the amplification is high, the "gain" is high; if we want to decrease the amplification, we "turn down the gain." In the strict sense, the attenuator is not a gain control. The gain control is the knob that adjusts the sensitivity of the amplifier and, as such, is sometimes labeled "sensitivity." Then again, some manufacturers label it "gain," and others label the attenuator "gain." Confusing, isn't it? To try to bring some order to this mess we shall define **gain** as the intensity of the echo signal presented to the display system: A Gain Control is any control which regulates this intensity. Under this definition there may be more than one knob which qualifies as the gain control. As we have seen, the attenuator definitely is a gain control. If the machine has a knob to adjust the amplifier, usually called "sensitivity," this also is a gain control. By adjusting either one we will affect the overall gain of the scanner. (The trend in most late model scanners is to refer to the attenuator as the "gain." Some scanners no longer have sensitivity controls on the front of the machine.) Now, back to our "SuperSon."

When an echo is received by the transducer crystal a very short oscillating voltage is produced. This is just the reverse of the transmitting process. The echo strikes the crystal and deforms it slightly; since the echo has the form of a sine wave, the deformations in the crystal will have the form of a sine wave, and the resulting electric voltage will also have the form of a sine wave. This is a happy circumstance because we are already used to thinking of sound in terms of sine waves and so we can just continue to use this pattern even though we are dealing with an electric signal instead of the actual echo.

Figure 3–2 shows the electric voltage pattern of a typical echo. Notice the sine wave form of the voltage. This echo was produced by a steel ball and so is quite loud; its maximum voltage is approximately 3.5 volts. This corresponds to the amplitude of an echo from soft tissue and bone. Most of the echoes from soft tissue inter-

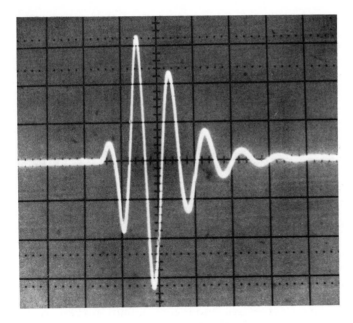

Figure 3–2. The electric signal generated by a returning echo has the form of a sine wave. This is the actual electric signal produced by an echo from a steel ball in water. The vertical axis is voltage (0.5 volt/division) and the horizontal axis is time (0.5 μsec/division). This is a very "loud" echo, comparable in magnitude to the echo from a soft tissue-bone interface. Notice that the transducer damping quickly suppresses the echo.

faces are 40 to 60 decibels softer and generate voltages in the range of one to 100 millivolts. Therefore it is necessary to amplify them before they can be sent to the display system.

This type of oscillating electric wave is also known as a radio frequency wave (abbreviated r.f. wave). To amplify such a wave will obviously require an r.f. amplifier. Fortunately many different types of r.f. amplifiers are available so we don't have to build one or know how it works; we'll just install a high quality one in our machine. It is important that we have a high quality amplifier so that it will be able to pick up the very tiny signals from the very weak echoes and amplify them without distorting them.

TIME COMPENSATED GAIN (TCG)

If there were no attenuation of the ultrasound beam in tissue, a simple r.f. amplifier would be adequate for our scanner. However, as we saw in Chapter 1, the beam is attenuated by approximately one decibel per centimeter per MegaHertz. This means that the echo from an interface will become weaker, the further the interface is located from the transducer.

Figure 3–3 illustrates a hypothetical scanning situation. A 2 MHz ultrasound beam is scanning a homogeneous tissue which has the same attenuation coefficient

as human soft tissue (1 dB/cm/MHz). There are only three interfaces in our hypothetical tissue; one is located 3 centimeters from the transducer, the second 6 centime-

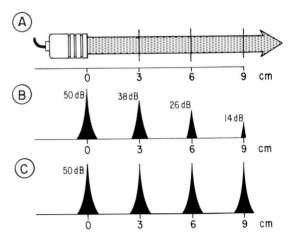

Figure 3–3. Echoes from deep interfaces are attenuated to a greater extent than echoes from near interfaces.

A, A 2 MHz ultrasound beam is directed through three interfaces located 3, 6, and 9 centimeters from the transducer. Each of these interfaces is the same and would give rise to a 50 dB echo if there were no attenuation of the beam.

B, Because of attenuation the echoes become progressively weaker. This line shows the amplitude of the echoes as they are received by the transducer.

C, To compensate for the loss of echo amplitude, TCG is used. TCG amplifies the deeper echoes more than the near echoes and restores each echo to its original 50 dB.

ters from the transducer, and the third is located at 9 centimeters. All three of these interfaces have the same acoustic impedance mismatch; that is, they would all give rise to the same amplitude echo if they were located the same distance from the transducer. However, since the interfaces are at different depths they will not give rise to echoes of equal amplitude because the echo from the deeper interfaces will be attenuated to a greater extent than the echo from the closest interface. Now suppose that, in the absence of any attenuation, this interface would yield an echo of 50 decibels. What amplitude echo will be received from the interfaces at 3, 6, and 9 centimeters? Since we are using a 2 MHz beam the attenuation will be: 2 MHz × 1 dB/cm/MHz = 2 dB/cm. The echo from the interface at 3 centimeters will have traveled 6 centimeters overall (3 going and 3 returning) and will have been attenuated: 6 cm × 2 dB/cm = 12 dB. Similarly, the echoes from the interfaces at 6 and 9 centimeters will have traveled 12 and 18 centimeters and will have been attenuated 24 and 36 decibels respectively. Thus the echoes received from these three interfaces would be (50−12)=38, (50−24)=26, and (50−36)=14 decibels.

Notice that although attenuation is dependent on frequency and distance, it does not depend on the basic amplitude of the echo. Weak and strong echoes will be attenuated the same amount. In the example of Figure 3–3 the attenuation is the same whether the original echo had an amplitude of 50 decibels or 36 decibels. (If the original echo indeed had an amplitude of 36 decibels, what would be the amplitude of the received echo from the interface at 9 centimeters? Could we detect this echo? Read on for the answer.)

Since attenuation depends only on distance and frequency, it is possible for us to compensate for this loss of amplitude by using our amplifier. All we need to do is to amplify echoes more if they come from a greater distance. Consider again the echoes in Figure 3–3, line B. Now we know that each of these echoes is supposed to have an amplitude of 50 decibels. Yet the received echoes had amplitudes of 38, 26, and 14 decibels. This means we must amplify the echo at 3 centimeters by 12 decibels, the one at 6 centimeters by 24 deci-

bels, and the one from 9 centimeters by 36 decibels. If we do that then all three echoes will emerge from the amplifier with an amplitude of 50 decibels (Figure 3–3, line C), and we will have corrected for attenuation. (How would this work if the original echo were 36 decibels? Pretty well, for the 3 and 6 centimeter interfaces; the echoes from these would be restored to their original 36 decibels. However, the echo from 9 centimeters was attenuated to 0 decibels and hence was never detected by the transducer. Thus there is no way we can amplify it and this echo would remain undetectable.)

This concept of correcting for attenuation using differential amplification is known as **time compensated gain** or **TCG**. The "time" refers to the fact that the amplifier automatically increases the gain as a function of time. But time is the same as distance in ultrasound. (Remember way back when we met the man who measured canyons by shouting across them? He repainted his watch face so that it read in distance instead of time.) Therefore, TCG really stands for distance compensated gain.

We are all ready to add TCG to our amplifier but how should we set it up? What rate of compensation should we use? If we knew that only a 2.25 MHz transducer was going to be used, then we could set it for the average attenuation which is: 2.25 MHz × 1 dB/cm/MHz = 2.25 dB per centimeter. However, this would not work so well with a 1.6 MHz or a 5.0 MHz transducer. It also might not work well with a 2.25 MHz transducer if the attenuation were much different from average. For instance, a cirrhotic liver has a very high attenuation and would require more compensation than average. A pregnant uterus has less than average attenuation and would need yet another setting. The obvious solution is to allow the ultrasonographer to select the TCG which is appropriate for the scanning situation. We shall put on a control which allows the TCG to be varied over as wide a range as possible; when the TCG control is turned up the differential amplification will be increased; when it is turned down it will be decreased. Figure 3–4 illustrates how this control affects the overall amplification or gain.

(*Advanced study department:* The TCG amplifier—which is usually part of the r.f.

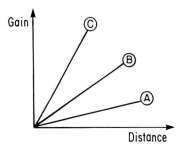

Figure 3-4. The amount of TCG can be varied to suit scanning needs. Three different settings are illustrated. The vertical axis shows the amount of gain and the horizontal axis shows the distance from the transducer.

A, A low TCG setting such as 0.8 dB/cm.

B, A higher setting such as 1.6 dB/cm.

C, A high setting, nearly 2.25 dB/cm.

The slope of the TCG line can be changed with a control on the scanner.

amplifier — is the most important single element of the sounder since it is the capacity of the TCG which limits the overall sensitivity of the ultrasound scanner. It is difficult and expensive to make a TCG with a range of more than 30 to 50 decibels. This is sufficient for echocardiography and echoencephalography in which the distances aren't great and the relative amplitudes of the echoes aren't very important, but in gray-scale abdominal scanning the limited range of the TCG can be a problem. The most common scanning frequency is 2.25 MHz. An interface only 10 centimeters deep [not at all uncommon in abdominal work] would need 45 decibels of TCG to avoid distortion. Some scanners simply aren't capable of producing this and hence they cannot record weaker echoes from these distances. When a 5 MHz transducer is used the TCG requirements are immense; 50 decibels at 5 centimeters. Usually TCG is added to the baseline amplification, which must be capable of 60 decibels to record the range of normal echoes. This means the total range of the amplifier should be on the order of 110 to 120 decibels. Continued improvements are being made in amplifiers but they represent a limiting factor in the sensitivity of ultrasound scanners. We should also notice that the TCG requirements are independent of transducer performance. That is, even if the transducer were perfect — a tightly focused beam with no loss of intensity due to dispersion — TCG would be necessary since attenuation is caused by the tissue itself. In practice, transducers are not perfect and the beam tends to be weaker in the far field, adding an even greater burden on the TCG amplifier.)

SPECIAL GAIN CONTROLS

As long as we are fiddling around with the gain we should consider adding some options to our machine which are sometimes found on commercial scanners. Every scanner has a TCG. Some also have a **near gain suppression.** As the name suggests, this control suppresses the amplification in the near field, usually the first 1 or 2 centimeters. It works just the reverse of the TCG. This is sometimes desirable because the near field echoes are usually quite strong (for two reasons: first, they are attenuated less, and second, they are frequently loud, specular echoes from the skin and body wall). Also, artifacts are more common in the near field (see Chapter 5 for more discussion of artifacts). Therefore, some ultrasonographers prefer to suppress the echoes for the first few centimeters. This is quite useful in echocardiography but we do not recommend its use in abdominal and pelvic scanning. We will not put a near gain suppression control on our "SuperSon." (We will go into the reasons for this in Chapter 6.)

Another popular control is the **reject.** This allows the ultrasonographer to select a level below which echoes will not be amplified. Another way of saying this is that an echo must have a certain minimum amplitude before it will be processed by the amplifier. The reject knob selects this level. The purpose of this control is to eliminate a lot of low level echoes and electronic noise which would otherwise clutter up the picture. As the reject control is turned up the weakest signals are eliminated. (A scratch filter on a stereo does much the same thing for high frequency noise on the record.) Unfortunately the reject will eliminate real echoes as well as noise; therefore, we do not think it has much use in abdominal scanning. We prefer to record all the echoes and then make a decision as to what is noise and what is real. Echocardiographers find the reject useful for their work but for abdominal and pelvic scanning: "reject the reject." (Bi-stable scanners have an inherent reject mechanism in the display system; this is one of the disadvantages of bi-stable scanning.)

Finally, some machines have replaced the simple TCG with a series of individual controls for various depths. This allows greater flexibility in setting the TCG since, instead of setting just the rate of TCG, the ultrasonographer can actually set the value of the gain at each centimeter of depth. Sounds great, huh? Well, it does add some flexibility but it also means that when you want to change the TCG you have to change a whole lot of controls instead of just one, and we are not sure whether that disadvantage makes the greater flexibility worth it. Each individual can decide this for himself, but we prefer the single TCG control for our "SuperSon."

SIGNAL PROCESSING

Now we have our amplified echoes which have been corrected for attenuation by the TCG. But they still look like Figure 3–2, a sine wave. We must do some processing so that the signal will be suitable for our display system.

First we must get rid of the negative component of the signal (the part below the base line) since display systems cannot work with negative signals. Therefore, we will send the signal through a circuit which eliminates the negative portion. This is known as **demodulation**. The only difference between the original and the demodulated signal is that the bottom parts of the sine waves have been cut off. (We could also just fold this bottom part over so that it was superimposed on the top but this doesn't have any practical advantage and is not done much.) Figure 3–5 shows the signal before and after demodulation.

The demodulated signal has two or three peaks and we must replace these with a

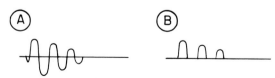

Figure 3–5. The echo signal must be demodulated before it can be sent to the display system.

A, The signal before demodulation.

B, The demodulated form. The negative components have been removed.

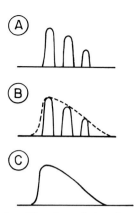

Figure 3–6. The demodulated signal consists of two or three peaks which must be converted to a single peak. This is done by electronically drawing an envelope over the peaks.

A, The demodulated signal.

B, An "envelope" is drawn over the peaks.

C, The final signal form. This process is known as *detecting* the signal.

single peak; otherwise the display system might think it was two or three different echoes. This is sometimes called **detecting** the signal. It is accomplished by a process known as "enveloping." A circuit draws an "envelope" over the tops of the waves, as illustrated in Figure 3–6.

The form of the echo, after enveloping, is known as a **video** form. This is in contrast to the sine wave forms with which we have been working up to now. The echo signal could be sent to the display system in this form, but most manufacturers refine it further to change the appearance of the final picture. Figure 3–7 illustrates some of the more common forms of signal processing.

The problem with the video form is that it is rather long and does not have a very sharp peak. This means it will yield a fairly fat dot with fuzzy edges when displayed on an oscilloscope or TV monitor. Also, the peak of the video form is not at the beginning of the echo, which is where the interface is actually located. Because of these difficulties with the video form, some type of electronic manipulation is generally applied to "improve" the shape of the signal. The first of these is differentiation.

As shown in Figure 3–7, this gives a much sharper peak at the very onset of the echo. It also gives a negative peak in the second half of the echo, but this can easily be filtered out and not sent to the display system. If differentiation is used, the dis-

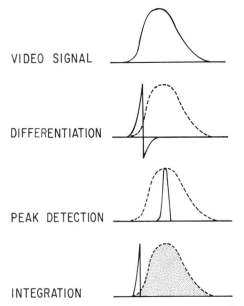

VIDEO SIGNAL

DIFFERENTIATION

PEAK DETECTION

INTEGRATION

Figure 3–7. There are many ways of modifying the video signal to change the appearance of the final image. A few of the more common processes are shown here. Different manufacturers use different types of signal processing.

play form is often referred to as "leading edge display." This form is commonly used for bi-stable scanning because it gives a sharp, narrow echo. It is less popular for gray-scale, however, because it does not give a very good representation of the amplitude of the echo.

The next type of electronic trickery is peak detection, a method whereby the maximum height or "peak" of the video form is measured and a narrow electric spike with this height is substituted for the video form. The spike can be located at either the beginning of the echo or at its peak. Peak detection gives a narrow signal and consequently a well-defined dot on the display monitor while preserving the amplitude information better than the differentiated wave form.

Amplitude data are even better preserved if integration, another form of electronic manipulation, is used. In this method the area underneath the video form is measured and a narrow spike, the height of which is proportional to this area, is substituted for the video form. The louder echoes obviously have larger areas than the softer echoes and will yield taller spikes.

It is possible to mix these manipulations, and there are other variations used by some manufacturers so that the final signal form can be somewhat different from machine to machine. There is no objective way of deciding what form of signal processing gives the "best" image, and the ultrasonographer will have to look at the pictures from various manufacturers to see which is most pleasing to his eye. Currently available scanners range from those which maintain a fairly sharp spike (and consequently a fairly sharp dot on the monitor) to those which deliberately "smooth" the edges of the spikes so that the dots on the monitor will blend into one another. The former give a rather "grainy" image, but the individual echoes can be clearly seen; the latter give a very uniform and smooth picture which more closely resembles a photograph, but it is more difficult to pick out the individual echoes and define tissue boundaries.

We prefer the "grainy" approach, but this is probably because we have done most of our work on this type of machine and feel more comfortable with it. Excellent clinical results can be obtained with any of the currently available gray-scale scanners. (For our "SuperSon" we shall incorporate both types of signal processing with a switch which will allow changing from one type to another as the whim strikes us.)

VIDEO AMPLIFIERS

Now that we have our echo signals demodulated, detected, and processed, we are ready to send them to the display system. Unfortunately, our sounder and transducer are more sensitive than any of the presently available display systems. We are picking up echoes with an amplitude range of at least 60 decibels, and, because we are using very sophisticated electronic circuitry in our sounder, we have managed to preserve this entire 60 decibel range during amplification and signal processing. Alas, the available display systems cannot handle this much information. The best quality cathode ray oscilloscopes can accept only about 25 decibels of data; scan converters are even more limited: the range of signals they can use is only 20 decibels.

We must somehow "compress" our 60 decibels of data down to the 20 or 25 decibels which our display system can make use of. As we will be using a scan converter for a display system, we really have an upper limit of 20 decibels with which to work. There are several types of amplifiers which can do this sort of thing for us. They go under various names, the most common being "logarithmic." They all effectively perform the same function; they take a large input range and compress it to a narrow output range. We want one which will take 60 to 80 decibels of input and yield 20 decibels of output.

Since this amplifier is being used on the signal when it is in the video wave form, it is known as a video amplifier. In addition to compressing the signals down to the 20 decibels, it will also adjust their intensity so that they will fit into the display system.

Well, the sounder portion of our "Super-Son" is complete. We can now proceed to the position monitor.

THE THREE MODES (A, M, and B)

Although we will be concerned primarily with B-mode scanning, it is useful to know about other modes as well.

A-mode (the "A" stands for amplitude) is the simplest. The signals from our basic sounder are in A-mode. Figure 3–8 shows this type of presentation. We can measure two parameters of the echoes: their distance from the transducer and their amplitude. The distance is usually displayed along a horizontal line on an oscilloscope. You will remember that distance and time are interchangeable in ultrasound because the beam is traveling at a constant rate (1540 meters/second or 1.54 millimeters/microsecond. Therefore, to get a display of distance, all we have to do is start the beam of an oscilloscope moving from left to right across the face of the scope at the same time we send out the pulse; we will adjust the speed of the oscilloscope beam so that it will travel 1 centimeter across the face of the scope in the same amount of time it would take the ultrasound beam to make the round trip to an interface 1 centimeter deep.

(*Quiz time:* How long is this? Hmmm! Let's see now. If the interface is 1 centimeter deep, the echo actually has to travel twice this distance to make the trip to the interface and return to the transducer, so we need to know how long it will take to go 2 centimeters. Two centimeters are 20 millimeters and the speed of sound is 1.54 millimeters per microsecond so the required time is 20 millimeters ÷ 1.54 millimeters/microsecond = 13.0 microseconds. Therefore we want the oscilloscope beam to travel 1 centimeter in 13 microseconds.)

Once the rate of the oscilloscope beam is set, we can just apply the signal from our sounder to it and cause the beam to be deflected upwards whenever an echo is received. This will generate a row of spikes on the oscilloscope screen, each spike cor-

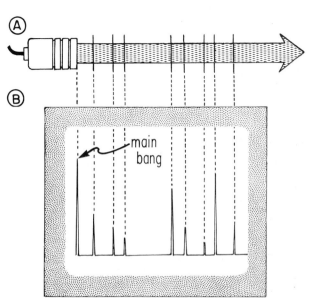

Figure 3–8. A-mode displays the echoes as a function of distance from the transducer.

A, An ultrasound beam passing through several interfaces.

B, The A-mode display of the echoes as they would appear on an oscilloscope. The oscilloscope trace starts with the "main bang," which corresponds to the transducer face. Each echo is displayed as a spike; the height of the spike is proportional to the amplitude of the echo. The distance from the main bang to the spike is proportional to the distance from the transducer to the interface.

responding to an echo. The distance between the spike and the start of the oscilloscope trace will be equal to the distance from the transducer to the interface which produced the echo, while the height of the spike will be proportional to the amplitude of the echo. The start of the oscilloscope trace is known, rather colorfully, as the "Main Bang."

The face of an oscilloscope is usually only 10 centimeters across; and, therefore, our display is limited to echoes within 10 centimeters of the transducer. The diameter of the abdomen is usually in the range of 20 to 30 centimeters and can be even greater in obese or pregnant patients. For abdominal work, therefore, we must decrease the scale of our display. This is a simple matter; if we have the oscilloscope beam travel one half as fast, then 1 centimeter on the scope will be equivalent to 2 centimeters in the patient. Even more useful is to have the beam travel one third as fast which will make 1 centimeter on the oscilloscope equal to 3 centimeters in the patient. This is known as scanning at a 3 to 1 ratio or 3 to 1 scale (sometimes written as 3:1). Ratios of 2:1 and 1:1 can also be useful if the part being scanned will fit on the display screen, and most scanners have a control which allows the operator to select the scale he wishes to use. These controls may offer scales as great as 4:1.

One problem with offering so many scales is that there needs to be some method of labeling each image with the scale used. This can be done by having the ultrasonographer write the scale on the back of the picture, but an even more useful method is to have a circuit which will generate reference spikes every centimeter. All modern scanners have such a circuit, known as the "scale markers" (naturally). This circuit is activated by pressing a control on the machine; the reference spikes will then be flashed on the picture and can be preserved for posterity.

A-mode is used in echoencephalography and echocardiography, but is only infrequently used in abdominal or pelvic scanning.

M-mode is basically A-mode with a minor variation. A-mode measures the position and amplitude of the echoes while M-mode records the position and the motion of the echo (the "M" stands for motion). To make M-mode we first start with the A-mode display. Each spike on the display is then replaced with a single dot. The brightness of the dot is made proportional to the amplitude of the echo. Now if all of the echo-producing interfaces are stationary the dots will remain stationary; but if one of the interfaces is moving, such as a heart valve or the wall of the aorta, the dot corresponding to that interface will also move. If the interface moves back and forth toward the transducer, the dot will also move back and forth toward the transducer.

To record this motion we can do one of two things: either we can slowly move the line of dots across the face of the oscilloscope from bottom to top or we can slowly run a photographic film or light-sensitive paper in front of the line of dots. Either method will produce the same image—a series of lines. Each line corresponds to an echo interface. Interfaces which are stationary will produce straight lines, while moving interfaces will produce wiggly lines. The wiggly line represents the motion of the echo with time. Figure 3–9 illustrates M-mode.

M-mode is used almost exclusively in echocardiography. It does, however, occa-

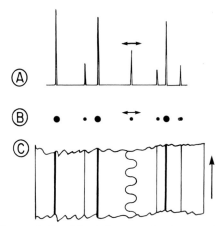

Figure 3–9. M-mode records the motion of echoes.

A, An A-mode display of echoes.

B, To obtain M-mode, the spikes are replaced with dots; the brightness of the dot is proportional to the height of the spike and the amplitude of the echo.

C, If an interface is moving the dot will also move and the motion of the dot can be recorded by running a light-sensitive paper in front of the display. Dots which are stationary produce straight lines while dots which move produce wiggly lines.

sionally crop up in abdominal work, usually to document the motion of the aorta or to record the fetal heartbeat.

B-mode is the mainstay of abdominal and pelvic ultrasonography. The "B" stands for brightness. This is not a particularly good description, and, if we were naming things over, we would call it P-mode to signify "picture." Figure 3–10 illustrates how this works.

First we start with the A-mode display and replace the spikes with dots, just as for M-mode. The brightness of the dot is made proportional to the amplitude of the echo; the louder the echo, the brighter the dot (this is where the name B-mode is derived). Now, instead of orienting the dots from left to right on the oscilloscope screen, we will have the line of dots oriented in the same direction that the transducer is pointing. When the transducer is moved, the line of dots corresponding to the echoes will move in the same direction. The display system will keep a record of all the dots so that, as the transducer is scanned across the patient, all of the echoes which are produced from the various interfaces will be displayed and recorded in the position from which they were produced. This concept is perhaps a little difficult to understand when put into words, but is actually quite easy to grasp visually. Reference to Figure 3–10 will probably be helpful and about two minutes of actual scanning will make the concept perfectly clear.

B-mode yields a two-dimensional picture of the area covered by the transducer. The amplitude information is maintained in the brightness of the dots. The picture actually represents a "slice" of the patient; the thickness of the slice will be equal to the width of the ultrasound beam. It is this ability to produce a two-dimensional image which makes B-mode scanning so useful to the ultrasonographer.

POSITION MONITOR

In order to maintain the proper orientation of the oscilloscope display, the transducer is attached to a series of hinged arms. These arms permit free movement in a single plane only. Figure 3–11 shows the hinged arm system. If the length of the arms and the angles between them are

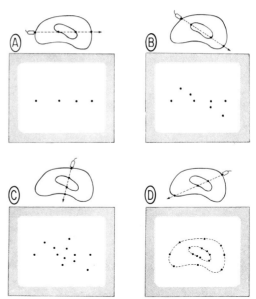

Figure 3–10. B-mode generates a "picture" of the area being scanned. The echo spikes in the A-mode presentation are replaced with dots; the brightness of the dot is proportional to the amplitude of the echo. Instead of orienting the dots on a horizontal axis, as is done in A-mode and M-mode, the dots are oriented in the same position and direction as the transducer. As the transducer is scanned across the patient, the dots will build up an image of the interfaces within the patient, as is illustrated in A to D. The top portion of each figure shows the orientation of the transducer on the patient, while the bottom portion of the figure shows the resulting image on the oscilloscope.

known, then it is possible to calculate the position and orientation of the transducer. (Those readers who get off on trigonometry are invited to derive the equations for solving this problem.) Since we hate trigonometry we shall install a small electronic calculating system in our position monitor to do this work for us.

The construction of this monitor and its arms is fairly straightforward but there are several things we need to watch out for. We must make certain that the arms are long enough to reach all the way around a large patient. In the past some commercial machines have had very short arms which necessitated scanning some patients in two stages, moving the scanning head in the middle of the scan. (The arms and their supporting structures are generally referred to as the "scanning head," by the way.)

It is also important that the arms be sta-

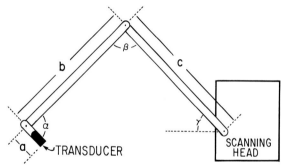

Figure 3–11. A hinged arm system limits transducer motion to a single plane. The position and orientation of the transducer within the plane can be calculated from the length of the arms, *a*, *b*, and *c*, and the angles between them, *α*, *β*, *γ*. An electronic system in the scanning head performs these calculations and sends the information to the display system.

ble with only minimum side-to-side motion. There is no way for our position monitor to compensate for side-to-side motion of the scanning plane; any such motion will result in a fatter "slice" of tissue being examined and, in effect, will decrease lateral resolution. In some commercial scanners this actually becomes the limiting factor in the lateral resolution of the entire scanner; if there is 2 centimeters of "play" in the scanning arms, then the resolution can be no better than 2 centimeters!

The entire scanning head should be as mobile as possible. As we shall see in later chapters, it is very important to scan patients in many planes. This is only practical if the scanning head can be easily moved to assume many different angles and heights. Our pet peeve with the manufacturers of ultrasound scanners is that they have not put much imagination into developing highly mobile and flexible scanning heads. (The only really satisfactory unit we have ever seen was developed in Europe and has never been marketed in this country.) We hope that this situation will be corrected in future machines.

Most scanners incorporate some sort of motor to move the scanning head a preselected distance along an axis at right angles to the scanning plane. This is quite useful in clinical scanning. It is also helpful to be able to disengage all locking mechanisms and freely move the head across the patient.

The angles between the arms are mea-

sured with electronic devices known as potentiometers. These potentiometers may drift out of adjustment and this will cause slight distortions in the B-mode image. Unfortunately, these distortions are usually so small that they cannot be readily recognized for what they are; instead they can be misinterpreted as distorted anatomy in the patient. The cure for this is simple. By scanning any of the various available test objects, these distortions become obvious and the appropriate adjustments can be made in the potentiometers. (These adjustments are quite simple and usually can be performed by an in-house service person.) A nationwide survey of ultrasound equipment sponsored by the American Institute of Ultrasound in Medicine showed that potentiometer misalignment was the most common malfunction of ultrasound scanners. It is, therefore, recommended that the potentiometers be checked at least every three months. (One manufacturer has replaced the potentiometers with "linear encoders," an electronic device said to be more stable. Only time will tell whether this works out in clinical use.)

The greatest difference in the various scanners on the market today is in the position monitor and scanning head system. We think that anyone contemplating purchase of a new piece of equipment should pay particular attention to the scanning head and how it works. It is especially important to try some actual scans with each of the machines under consideration; there is nothing more frustrating in day-to-day clinical ultrasound work than a scanning head mechanism with which the ultrasonographer is not comfortable. For our ideal "SuperSon" we shall design a featherweight arm system, precision balanced so that it floats over the patient's skin. The entire scanning head will be no larger than a bread box and will be motor driven in three directions, including the vertical. Scanning will be possible in any plane, including those parallel to the floor. The entire unit will be tastefully packaged in a brushed aluminum case with gold engraved "SuperSon-Alpha" on the front and an American flag on the back.

Now our position monitor is complete and we shall hitch it up to our sounder. We are ready to proceed to the final aspect of our scanner—the display system.

OSCILLOSCOPE DISPLAYS

The processed video signal from the sounder is integrated with the position monitor and then sent to the display system where is is converted to a visual form. This involves either an oscilloscope or a TV monitor. We shall consider the oscilloscope first.

An oscilloscope is a cathode ray tube. We do not want to get too involved with the physics of these devices and will consider only a couple of things. Cathode ray tubes consist of a gun which shoots a tiny beam of electrons at a phosphor target. When the electron beam strikes the target it causes the phosphor to glow and produces a small dot of light. The brightness of this dot is proportional to the intensity of the electron beam; if the beam is intense the spot will be brighter than if the beam is weak. Therefore we will feed the amplitude information in our video signal to the electron beam; the loud echo generates a high amplitude video signal which will produce an intense electron beam and consequently a bright dot on the phosphor screen. As we mentioned previously, the intensity of the dot can be varied only over a limited range, about 25 decibels in the highest quality scopes and 20 decibels or less in the average oscilloscope. (However, we took care of this by compressing the signal with our video amplifier.)

The electron beam is steered about the target by either electric plates or electromagnets (if plates are used the scope is said to be electrostatic; if electromagnets are used the scope is—what else?—electromagnetic). The time and position information in our signal will be fed to this steering mechanism, and this will assure that the electron beam is properly aimed so that the echoes will appear in the correct location. This aiming mechanism is quite precise in an oscilloscope, and very little distortion is introduced into the picture. As we shall see, a TV monitor has more distortion than an oscilloscope.

It is desirable to have the dots as small as possible because the resolution of the scope is inversely proportional to the dot size. This size varies with the quality of the oscilloscope and the type of phosphor. The most commonly used oscilloscopes have a diagonal screen measurement of 15 centimeters and a dot size of about .05 centime-

ter. The size of the dot ultimately limits the resolution of our scanner since it is obviously not possible to resolve two echoes if their dots overlap.

(We caught you dozing off there. It seems time to have a *short quiz* again. If the oscilloscope has a dot size of .05 centimeter, what is the theoretic resolution limit when the scope is scanning on a 1:1 scale? On a 3:1 scale? Let us consider the 1:1 scale first. This means that 1 centimeter on the scope is equal to 1 centimeter in the patient. Since the resolution on the scope is .05 centimeter, the resolution in the patient will be .05 centimeter or 0.5 millimeter. Now when we scan on a 3:1 scale everything is reduced in size so that 1 centimeter on the scope corresponds to 3 centimeters in the patient. Therefore .05 centimeter on the scope will be equivalent to .15 centimeter in the patient and the resolution limit will be 1.5 millimeters. This is poorer than the theoretic resolution limit imposed by the frequency of the transducer.)

The oscilloscope provides us with a convenient way of displaying the echoes but we need some method of storing them so we can see the entire scan picture at once. (The phosphor only produces a dot when the electron beam is actually hitting it.) There are two ways of doing this: film and storage oscilloscopes.

STORAGE OSCILLOSCOPES

It is possible to modify an oscilloscope so that it will "store" dots; that is, once a dot appears on the screen it remains there until erased by the operator. Such scopes are known as storage oscilloscopes. If such a scope is used, an entire picture of an ultrasound scan can be produced and held on the face of the target. The ultrasonographer can then view the picture, make a diagnostic decision, modify the scan, and photograph the image in a leisurely fashion.

Unfortunately, there are two serious problems with the storage oscilloscope which limit its usefulness in modern B-mode ultrasonography. First is dot size. The size of the dot on a storage scope is about twice as large as the dot would be on a non-storage scope. A typical average dot size is 0.1 centimeter which limits the resolution on a 3:1 scan to 3 millimeters as opposed to 1.5 mm on the non-storage unit. Also, as the scope ages, dot size increases; and resolution decreases even further. Although this imposes a theoretic limit on the usefulness of a storage oscilloscope, in clinical use the dot size does not seriously compromise the diagnostic quality of the image.

A greater difficulty is the bi-stable nature of the storage display. A dot on the storage scope is either "on" or "off" (bi-stable means existing in only two states). Therefore the amplitude information of the video signal cannot be directly displayed on a storage oscilloscope. This amplitude information will fall into one of two classes; either the echo will be sufficiently loud to trigger a dot or it will have insufficient intensity to generate a dot and nothing will be recorded. The level at which a dot will appear on a storage scope is known as the threshold of the scope. Any echo at or above threshold will produce the same size and brightness of dot. The final picture will have only two shades—black and white—no intermediate gray shades will be displayed. (It is possible to get gray-scale information from a storage oscilloscope, but it must be done indirectly. By starting the scan at very low gain only the very loudest echoes will be above the threshold of the scope; the picture produced at low gain will thus represent only these loud echoes. If the same scan is then repeated with the gain increased slightly, the next level of echoes will be above threshold and will be added onto the picture. This procedure—continually repeating the scan while slowly increasing the gain—will eventually give the ultrasonographer the complete amplitude information.)

It is clear that it would be preferable to have a display system which would enable us to preserve all of the amplitude information on a single image. There are two common methods of achieving this: standard oscilloscope with film and TV scan converters. Before we leave the subject of storage oscilloscopes and bi-stable scanning, however, we should acknowledge their importance in the history of abdominal ultrasound scanning. For several years this display system has been the mainstay of clinical ultrasound around the world; virtually all that is known about ab-dominal and pelvic ultrasound diagnosis was discovered and developed on bi-stable scanners; and, in the hands of an ultrasonographer skilled in its use, it can provide all of the diagnostic information that is available with the current gray-scale scanners. We shall discuss the topic of bi-stable scanning further in Chapter 12.

OSCILLOSCOPE-FILM COMBINATION

Gray-scale information can be produced if a standard oscilloscope, rather than a storage scope, is used and the image recorded on film. Film has several inherent advantages: a good range of gray, which is capable of reproducing all of the amplitude information on the oscilloscope, and high resolution, which will not degrade the image. Even the much-maligned Polaroid Type 107 film is capable of producing excellent images with a good gray scale.

There are two main disadvantages to the oscilloscope-film system: (1) The image cannot be seen until it is complete and the film has been developed. The ultrasonographer, therefore, cannot monitor the progress of the scan, and it is difficult to use any special techniques or concentrate on one particular area in the image. (2) Performing the scans is difficult because each area of the film should be exposed for the same amount of time. If the scanning motion is irregular or if compound scanning is used, the resulting image will be uneven and the shades of gray will have lost much of their meaning.

(Wait a minute! Someone is confused. Isn't film used to record most ultrasound images? All you need to do is push a button and the picture is taken, right? We are sorry for the confusion. Yes, indeed! Most final ultrasound images are recorded on film, but in these cases the film is used only to make a permanent record of the image on the display system. The film itself does not have anything to do with making the image and is not part of the display system. When film is used only to record an image which was produced some other way, the film is said to be **hard copy**. We shall discuss the different hard copy systems in Chapter 4. When film is used with an oscilloscope as part of the display system, the exposure technique is different.

The camera shutter is left open throughout the scan and the film exposed by the moving dots on the oscilloscope screen. In the early days of ultrasound this was known as scanning with the "open shutter technique." The image is not seen until the film is developed.)

A few ultrasonographers have been able to perfect the open shutter technique required for oscilloscope-film display work, but most of us find it extremely frustrating. The only consistently good scans with this system have been made with mechanically driven scanning heads. When coupled with a mechanical scanner, however, the images from oscilloscope-film displays are beautiful and clearly superior to images produced by scan converters.

The difficulties with storage oscilloscopes and oscilloscope-film combinations described above have made TV scan converters the most popular display system for current gray-scale scanners.

SCAN CONVERTERS AND TV MONITORS

Television scan converters have been around for more than 20 years (they were originally developed for the army by a Howard Hughes company) but have only recently been applied to ultrasound scanners. Every commercial scanner uses a scan converter and so this is one part of our "Super-Son" which we cannot alter. Still, we should know what this device is doing for us and what its limitations are.

Scan converters use a television monitor to produce the image. A TV monitor is similar in many ways to an oscilloscope. There is an electron gun which shoots a tiny electron beam toward a phospor target. When the beam hits the target it produces a small dot of light and the brightness of the dot is controlled by the intensity of the beam. However, the beam is not steered in the same manner as in an oscilloscope.

The electron beam in a TV starts at the upper left corner and sweeps horizontally across the screen from left to right until it reaches the far side. It then drops down slightly and makes another horizontal sweep just under the first. This process is repeated until the beam reaches the bottom of the screen; it then returns to the upper left corner and starts all over again. This process is analogous to the way we read the page of a book: we sweep our eyes across the top line of print, then return and read the second line and continue until we finish the entire page, then we start again at the top of the next page.

This scanning of the electron beam across the screen is standardized and internally controlled. Although there are several different TV formats, all ultrasound scanners use the standard American TV format (the same as commercial television). In this format the beam scans 525 horizontal lines and repeats this process 60 times per second. (Actually the beam scans every other line every 1/30 of a second; this reduces the flicker in the image.) We can see that the vertical (we will call it "up-and-down" to avoid confusion) resolution of a TV monitor is limited by the 525 scan lines available. Even if a larger screen face is used, there will still be only 525 lines of information. If you look closely at a TV picture you can see these lines; naturally they are easier to see on a larger screen than on a smaller one. It is difficult to predict how this will limit resolution on our scan since the spacing of the lines on the monitor will vary with respect to the scanning scale. We can examine a typical monitor, however, and get a rough idea of the resolution as it relates to our clinical scanning.

Virtually all of the commercial scanners utilize a 5-inch TV monitor for the hard copy system. Because of factors which need not concern us, these monitors cannot actually produce the theoretic 525 lines available. Instead they produce about 345 lines. When scanning on the 3:1 scale, 1 centimeter in the patient covers approximately 12 scan lines on the monitor and so the "up-and-down" resolution is approximately .83 millimeter.

Horizontal ("side-to-side") resolution is even harder to estimate. This is governed by how quickly the intensity of the electron beam can be changed. We must remember that the electron beam is scanning very rapidly, and if there is any delay in changing its intensity, the beam will have moved past the point where the dot should have been produced. The ability to change the beam rapidly depends on the quality of the electronics in the TV; high quality TV can do this very quickly and thus has good "side-to-side" resolution. Cheaper TV monitors have poorer resolution (this, of course, is hardly earthshaking news). The theoretic "side-to-side" resolution of the 5-inch monitor when used on the 3:1 scale is approximately 1.0 millimeter.

One problem with the TV monitor is distortion at the picture edges. It is not possible to produce a flat TV image which does not have distorted edges because the electron beam has to travel further to reach the edges than it does to reach the center of the picture and the slight delay causes the dot to be displaced a small amount. For this reason the ultrasonographer should try to keep his scans in the middle of the monitor, and no ultrasonic measurements should be made in the outer parts of the picture.

Another problem with TV monitors (and scan converters) is the limited range of brightness, about 20 decibels. This is poorer than a high quality oscilloscope. In addition, the brightness varies spontaneously unless expensive electronic supporting circuits are included. This causes the gray shades of the echoes to drift during the course of a day or even during a single scan. Fortunately, all the echoes change in the same direction, so the overall effect is only that the picture becomes lighter or darker. Still, this is annoying; it makes it difficult to couple a sensitive hard copy system to a TV monitor and makes the absolute intensity of any echo less reproducible. We hope equipment manufacturers will start including electronic circuits for controlling TV drift in their newer models (we will certainly include one in the "SuperSon").

The TV picture, however, does have some advantages. (1) There are brightness and contrast controls included in the monitor which permit altering the appearance of the final image. This may be helpful in distinguishing areas of similar echo density. (2) Videotape can be easily interfaced with the display system. (3) By changing the polarity of the video input the black and white areas can be interchanged. Thus, by merely flipping a switch, one can have black echoes on a white background or white echoes on a black background. (We are not sure whether this is a true advantage. Although it gives people something to talk and write about, it would be nice if a common standard were selected so that all images were presented the same way. Throughout this book we will use the convention of dark dots on a light background; thus a light gray dot represents a weak echo while a dark dot represents a loud echo.)

Now to the scan converter. The scan converter accepts the video output signal from the sounder, assigns a gray level to each echo, stores the information, and feeds it to the TV monitor. The actual operation of a scan converter is quite complicated, and it is capable of a great many manipulations of the image. We shall only take a superficial look at its insides.

It is perhaps simplest to think of a scan converter as a cross between a storage oscilloscope and a TV. It uses an electron gun which is scanned just as in a TV monitor. However, the target or screen is not a phosphor but a semiconductor. When the electron beam strikes the target it changes the electric charge on the semiconductor. The charge pattern on the target "stores" the image in a manner analogous to a storage oscilloscope. This stored charge pattern is then "read" by another electron beam and the output sent to the TV monitor.

There are several operations which can be performed on the stored image. The most important is assigning a shade of gray to each point on the target. This can be done rather arbitrarily. Most manufacturers have chosen to use between eight and ten different gray levels. This means that the final image, as it appears on the TV monitor, will be composed of eight to ten different shades of gray. It will be easiest to understand how this works by considering a specific example.

Let us suppose that, for our "SuperSon," we will use ten shades of gray. For convenience, we shall letter them in order with pure white being shade A and pure black being shade J. Shade B would be slightly darker than shade A, shade C slightly darker than shade B, etc. Next, we shall assign each of the echoes to one of the ten shades of gray. Now the sounder received echoes with a range of at least 60 decibels; the weakest echo had an amplitude of 1 decibel and the loudest an amplitude of 60 decibels. Since the scan converter can only accept echo signals over a range of 20

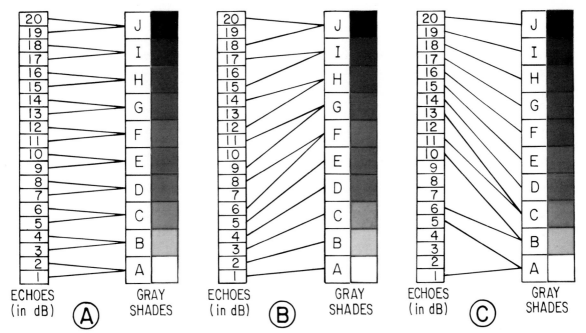

Figure 3–12.   Echoes can be assigned to shades of gray in many ways.

A, A uniform distribution; each shade of gray corresponds to 2 dB of echo amplitude.

B, A distribution which emphasizes the weak echoes; five shades of gray are assigned to the weakest 5 dB while the remaining five shades of gray are spread over 15 dB.

C, A distribution emphasizing the strong echoes; most of the gray shades are assigned to the six loudest echoes.

decibels we compressed the 60 decibels down to 20 decibels with our video amplifier so that we now have echo signals ranging from 1 to 20 decibels which we must assign to the shades of gray.

One way of doing this would be to divide the 20 decibels up in even steps; that is, 1 and 2 decibel echoes would be assigned to shade A, 3 and 4 decibels to shade B, 5 and 6 decibels to shade C, etc. We might also choose to distribute the gray shades unevenly. We could emphasize the soft echoes by assigning more shades of gray to the weak echoes. In that case we might have the 1 decibel echoes be gray shade A, the 2 decibel echoes gray shade B, the 3 decibel echoes shade C, the 4 decibel echoes shade D, and the 5 decibel echoes shade E. Echoes from 6 to 8 decibels would go to shade F, while 9 to 11 would be assigned shade G, 12 to 14 shade H, 15 to 17 shade I, and 18 to 20 shade J. Figure 3–12 shows some of the ways that the echoes can be matched to the shades of gray.

How do we go about assigning echoes to shades of gray? Quite simply, actually: the scan converter has a knob which controls the distribution of gray shades. Most manufacturers make this control available; it is usually called **enhance** or **contrast**. By altering the settings of this knob the scan image can be changed from one emphasizing dark gray shades to one with predominantly lighter shades. We do not feel that altering this control is useful and recommend that it be left alone. When this knob is moved the entire distribution of the gray scale is altered. Much of the potential value of gray-scale scanning is lost if the gray shades are constantly changed. The goal of gray-scale should be to obtain as reproducible an image as possible and fooling around with the enhance control is certain to destroy reproducibility. Therefore, set the enhance control in the middle of its range and do not touch it again.

You may have been wondering why only eight to ten shades of gray are used; why not use 20 shades and give each echo its own private gray tone? We do not have a satisfactory explanation. Some reasons which are given include: (1) "The human eye can only distinguish nine or ten shades of gray anyway." (This is not true. Most people can distinguish about 16 shades of gray if back illumination is used.) (2) "The image pattern is not improved by having more shades, because this would decrease the contrast of the image." (This may well be true.) (3) "The echo amplitude information is not so accurate or reproducible that it warrants using more shades—doing so would imply a precision to the image which is unjustified." (We are not sure we even understand this reasoning.) Whatever the reason, most commercial scanners generate only eight to ten gray levels.

Another image manipulation which is built into the scan converter is magnification. It is possible to magnify a portion of the stored image up to six times. This permits "zooming" in on a small part of the scan and "blowing it up." The value of this feature is debatable. Equipment manufacturers and many ultrasonographers think it is very useful. We are not so enthusiastic. The "zoom" does not improve the resolution; it simply magnifies the picture and the same thing can be done with a magnifying glass. In fact, to our eyes, resolution appears to be decreased when the picture is enlarged with the zoom control. We recommend setting the zoom control at zero magnification and not using it. If a larger picture is needed the scan should be performed on a different scale, such as 2:1 or 1:1. This will not only give a larger picture but will also improve resolution. (One redeeming feature of the zoom, however, is the capability of moving the picture about the screen with a joystick. This permits a region of particular interest to be centered on the monitor.)

The scan converter has some shortcomings. (1) The storage target is a matrix with 1000 elements on a side. In actual use the matrix is not that fine since electronic noise and electron beam tracking errors cause some overlap. The result is that the converter has a limited resolution. The resolution of the scan converter, however, is better than the resolution of the TV monitor; and, therefore, the scan converter will not degrade our picture significantly. (2) There is some drift and variation of the image, but again this is less serious than in the TV monitor. (3) When a scan is being performed and the storage target written upon, flickering lines appear across the image, causing a Venetian blind effect. Although

this is annoying when first encountered, it is quite easy to get used to and does not cause any difficulties in clinical scanning. The latest scan converters have eliminated this flicker. (4) Scan converters need periodic adjustment to maintain good differentiation of gray levels; along with the potentiometers in the scanning arms this is the component of the scanner which requires the most service.

Despite these minor problems, the scan converter remains the most useful overall method of displaying gray-scale B-scans. Before its introduction, gray-scale scanning was confined to the research laboratory and not practical for the general ultrasonographer. We shall incorporate a scan converter as the display system in our "Super-Son."

There is one final item we must take care of before our display system is ready for use. We must have some mechanism to prevent "overwriting." If we were to hold the transducer in one spot on the patient, the echo signals would keep piling up on the storage target until it was saturated. Similarly, if we scan over an area more than once the echoes from that area will be written on the storage target more than once. Suppose we are dealing with an echo from the liver with an amplitude of 8 dB. If we scan that echo once an 8 dB signal will be written on the storage target. Now if we pass the sound beam over this echo again, another 8 dB signal will be written on top of the original signal (we say the original signal has been overwritten). The storage target will now have the equivalent of a 16 dB signal instead of the correct 8 dB signal.

Two mechanisms are employed to prevent overwriting. First, the scan converter incorporates a "comparator" circuit. Before any signal is written on the storage target this circuit will compare the signal with what is already on the target. If the target already contains a signal of equal or greater strength, the new signal will not be written. If the target does not contain a signal of equal strength, the signal will be sent to the target in place of the signal which was previously there. What this means is that instead of adding signals together on the target the comparator circuit will write only the loudest available signal. Thus, if an area is scanned twice, the echoes from the second scan will only be written if they are of greater amplitude than the original echoes.

The second protection against overwriting involves a circuit which senses whether the transducer is in motion. This circuit allows the sounder to generate pulses only while the transducer is being moved. When the transducer is stationary, no pulses are generated. This mechanism prevents overwriting from the transducer being held in one spot. (It sometimes gives rise, however, to annoying skip areas when the transducer is being moved very slowly.)

THE COMPLETE SCANNER

It is time to break out the beer and pretzels. We have finished our basic scanner. There are several "options" we could add such as an alphanumeric display, digital readout of echo amplitudes, EKG gating, electronic depth measurement, and so on. Most commercial machines have several of these features. All have their uses, but they are not necessary for adequate clinical ultrasonography. We shall not discuss them in any detail; each ultrasonographer can experiment on his own to see whether there is a use for these options in his practice.

Chapter 4

LABORATORY
ORGANIZATION

A chapter devoted to the set-up of the ultrasound laboratory may seem a bit humdrum now that you have spent all that time with the mysterious workings of the scanning instruments themselves; but before you give up too quickly, let us assure you that the design and organization of the laboratory are fundamental to the smooth integration of ultrasound into the day-to-day operation of a busy medical center. This may not be apparent as a program gets under way because it is always easy to work in a case or two here or there as things get started. As the caseload builds, however, good organization is vital; therefore, it is best to start out on the right track and set everything up so that a full ultrasound schedule can be accommodated when the time to do so comes.

LABORATORY SET-UP

Let us consider the problem of laboratory set-up. First, there is the matter of the laboratory or examining room itself. (It is not clear why ultrasound facilities are usually referred to as "laboratories," a word which conjures up visions of guinea pigs and experimental procedures. Ten years ago this term was appropriate; but now the clinical value of ultrasound scanning is well enough established that it is—or should be—available in every well-equipped hospital. The terminology is well entrenched, however; and we will not take it upon ourselves to root it out.) How much space is really necessary and how should it be set up? Obviously, we would all like as much space as possible. As it works out, most ultrasound labs begin as converted closets, dressing rooms, or storage areas. If the ultrasound lab is to function efficiently, however (and if the opportunity to plan its construction from the start is presented), an

area of at least 300 square feet should be sought. We are talking about total space measuring 15 feet by 20 feet, for example. Put in a frame of reference known more or less to us all, this is about 5 feet longer than a modern diagnostic X-ray room. In even simpler terms, if you live in an older house, it is about the same size as an average bedroom; in a newer dwelling it would be the size of the family room (all of which goes to show how our emphasis has changed over the years). The entrance should allow easy access for a stretcher. In addition to the 300 square feet there should be nearby dressing and waiting rooms, as well as toilet and handwashing facilities for patients' use. Storage for linen, film, and other supplies in the examining area itself is a must. The optimum set-up is one in which the scanning area is actually separate from the support area, so that review of studies and x-rays as well as consultation can be carried out beyond earshot and view of the patient (Fig. 4–1).

It is impossible to overestimate the importance of finding a comfortable scanning table with a firm but soft mattress. After all, patients will be lying on it for as long as an hour, and you want them to be able to lie still. Be certain also that the examining table is wide enough so that the patient can turn on his side without fear of falling off. We rescued an old physical therapy table from storage and bought a four-inch foam mattress from a mail-order supplier. It was very inexpensive; and our patients often tell us how comfortable it is to lie there while being scanned, especially in comparison with the hard top of an ordinary X-ray table.

Give yourself enough room so that you can roll a stretcher into the scanning room without obstruction and examine the patient on that if need be. We find it easy to move our table aside to bring in a stretcher,

42

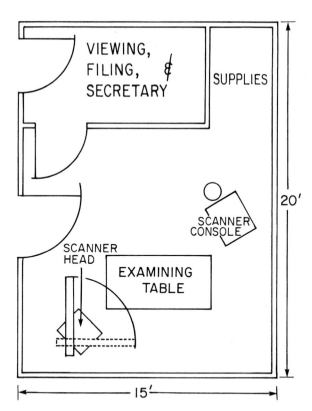

Figure 4-1. A comfortable ultrasound laboratory should have at least 300 square feet of floor space. This is an idealized floor plan for a functional laboratory—many equally good variations can be designed, but the important elements are included here.

and it certainly saves time (and your back) if patients do not have to be moved from the stretcher. Make certain that there is enough room to move the scanning head of your instrument easily from longitudinal to transverse position. (Usually the manufacturer will be able to provide information about the area needed for this.) You will also need enough room for a table to keep beside the scanner so that there is a place to put out your scans for review while the scanning is in progress. This is not so important when X-ray film is used for hard copy; but if Polaroid is your recording medium, you will want space for labeling, sorting, and reviewing. We have found an old hospital overbed table ideal for this. Its height can be varied to accommodate both short and tall ultrasonographers, and it can be rolled over the patient's legs for very convenient access to the sterile trays during biopsies and amniocenteses. If its appearance offends your aesthetics when it is first dragged out of the hospital's storage area, it is no trick at all to refinish it to match the laboratory or your personal tastes.

We have occasionally found a need for oxygen and suction and recommend that

these be included in any laboratory being constructed; portable oxygen and suction can be more efficiently supplied in an older converted laboratory. Extra electrical outlets are also essential; additional electronic gear is always a possibility in a fast-growing science, and there is the inevitable tiny newborn who needs a heated incubator (the batteries in which always seems to be low).

Overhead lights pose a problem. Viewing the television screens of the gray-scale scanners or the cathode ray tubes of the bistable ones is more comfortable, we find, in subdued light. For this reason, variable intensity lighting is desirable. A somewhat lower light is used when scanning, while bright light is available when a biopsy or amniocentesis is being done. There is not much that can be done about this when you have to make do with the converted closet; but, again, if you are planning a new laboratory, keep it in mind. (We find that everyone seems to look better in the dimmed light of the scanning room—technologists, physicians, even the patients. Now we know why the light level in cocktail lounges is always subdued.)

You will certainly need a telephone; and,

if your department has an intercom system, a station in the ultrasound lab is very helpful. Frequently ultrasound patients will be having conventional X-ray studies following the ultrasound scans; and, for this reason, the ability to communicate with other parts of the department is very valuable.

A few more items which are important: large wastebaskets to take care of Polaroid debris, stepstool (for getting on and off the examining table), I.V. pole, a bulletin board, an X-ray view box, and an inexhaustible supply of towels and linen.

SCHEDULING

Once an ultrasound program is initiated, it will not be long until it will be necessary to schedule patients in advance. As we mentioned above, often patients will be having conventional radiologic studies at the same time, and other patients will go immediately to physician appointments at which the ultrasound data will be important. Scheduling makes it necessary to have a secretary available to answer the telephone and to make the appointments, because the busy ultrasound technologist will not have time to interrupt work for such matters. Obviously, telephone scheduling is almost mandatory for out-patients. In-patients can usually be managed by the ordinary mechanism of sending request-for-examination slips to the ultrasound lab. The timing on in-patients is also usually somewhat more flexible.

There are some fundamental rules about patient preparation which influence scheduling, and we will go into them first. To begin, barium and gas in the intestine are mortal enemies of the ultrasonographer, because they prevent transmission of sound and usually make it impossible to get a satisfactory study. For this reason, any ultrasound scan of the abdomen should be done before barium is given (either by mouth or enema) and should not be scheduled within 12 hours of proctoscopy or sigmoidoscopy, because the large bowel will often be filled with air during these examinations. Iodinated contrast agents used to visualize the kidneys or gallbladder (Renografin, Hypaque, Conray, Telepaque, and the like) do not interfere with ultrasound. Also, when examining the struc-

tures in the upper abdomen, such as the pancreas or the gallbladder, it is preferable to have the patient fasting. By the same token, when scanning the pelvis for either a gynecological or an obstetrical problem, it is absolutely essential to have the urinary bladder full. It is clear, then, that scheduling will take some planning if things are to move along efficiently.

We have found that, on the average, a general abdominal examination cannot be done practically in less than 45 minutes. Much of this time will be spent on chores other than actual scanning. In-patients have to be called from their floors, the patients have to be brought into the room and put onto the examining table, the hard copies have to be made and identified, all the red-tape activity (billing, making out film jackets and other records, for example) has to be taken care of, the physician-ultrasonographer has to check the findings and may have to scan a bit as well, the patient has to be taken out of the room, and the linen has to be changed. On top of all of this are delays which arise because patients are late. (In our case, this is more of a problem with in-patients; our out-patients, many of whom travel long distances over very snowy roads in winter, are almost always on time.) We have a technical aide, and this helps with many of these activities; but this means employing another warm body and increases the overhead. It is certainly worthwhile to provide such supporting help, however, once the level of work climbs above four or five patients per day.

Bearing all of this in mind, then, there are some general rules for scheduling which will help make things go more smoothly (Table 4–1). We begin the day with in-patients who are to have both abdominal scans and a gastrointestinal barium study such as an upper GI series or a barium enema. We do this because these patients are fasting anyway and are gener-

TABLE 4–1. Rules for Scheduling

1—In-patient abdomens having barium studies first in morning
2—Out-patient abdomens having barium studies follow in-patients in morning
3—Obstetrical and gynecological patients in late morning and early afternoon
4—In-patient abdomens in late afternoon

ally readily available to us. We then schedule out-patients in a similar category. Out-patients might find it a bit difficult to get in to an early 8:00 A.M. appointment, but the need to have them fasting makes it desirable to examine them relatively early in the day so as to keep things from being any more unpleasant than necessary. By this time in the day, say 9:30 to 10:00 A.M., it is often necessary to break into the schedule to examine a gallbladder which has failed to visualize with the oral contrast agent. This type of study generally does not take 45 minutes and can usually be completed in 20 to 30 minutes, so that they are not difficult to accommodate.

We follow the early morning abdominal scanning with obstetrical cases. Usually these are out-patients, and we see them through the mid-portion of the day (late morning and early afternoon). These studies often go significantly more quickly than the 45-minute time slots we have provided for them, and this allows us to squeeze in those gallbladders we mentioned earlier and an emergency case or two that we have not scheduled. Remember, a full urinary bladder is a must for most obstetrical and all gynecological scanning. If your patient urinates, it will be an hour or two before her bladder will be full enough to try again, even if you have her drink several glasses of liquid. We have found it easier to allow our patients to empty their bladders after getting up in the morning, and then not urinate again until the study has been performed. Here is an area where a little planning is required in each case. When the appointment is made, the patients are instructed to empty their bladders about two hours before their appointment and at the same time to drink several glasses of water (or for that matter, any liquid—coffee, tea, whatever they like). From that time until we have examined them, they must hold on. (One common mistake: once the patient has suffered for an hour or two riding over bumpy roads to get to us, she makes it to the hospital with a full bladder and decides she is now home free. Before coming to the ultrasound lab, she asks for directions to the ladies' room and relieves herself.) If the importance of the full bladder is made clear to the patient when the appointment is made, things will go much more smoothly for everyone.

We schedule a somewhat longer period of time (1 to 1 1/2 hours) for obstetrical patients who are to have an amniocentesis, because the procedure itself takes considerably longer. Such patients are seen at the end of the morning when the extra time spent with them will not slow things greatly. In-patient obstetrical and almost all gynecological cases we do in the afternoon unless there is a pressing reason to get at them earlier. The in-patients generally do not have other demands on their time, and they are available when it is most convenient for us.

The odds and ends of scanning (thyroid, testicle, occasional chest) we schedule in the afternoon, as they usually do not require preparation and fit in best with other clinical activities such as physician appointments, house officer availability to help with procedures such as thoracentesis, and absence of conflict with other tests.

Finally, we save some in-patients' abdominal scanning for late in the day. We do this for several reasons. If out-patients fail to keep appointments or the studies go more quickly than expected, the in-patients can always be moved up. Moreover, the patients can have breakfast and fast at lunch, so they are not uncomfortable all day. In this way we can speed up the morning work by examining some of those patients who will have to have barium studies later.

Our schedule will not be satisfactory for everyone, but the principles are sound. It is important to maintain flexibility because unavoidable and unpredictable emergencies crop up every day and have to be managed. With a busy practice in ultrasound, we have found that adhering to the old adage, "Don't put off 'til tomorrow what you can do today," has helped us keep abreast of the demands placed upon our services; and our ability to accommodate referring physicians' needs without delay has enabled us to build our practice quickly. Almost always we find that the schedule cannot be made up entirely until the beginning of each day's work; therefore, the technologist should arrange to arrive 15 minutes or so early so that the schedule for that day can be finalized.

Between the hours of 8:00 A.M. and 4:30 P.M., we find that we can comfortably examine nine patients per scanning room. Try as we might, we have found it difficult to expand our workload beyond this level, and we doubt that good work can be carried on if the number exceeds this. We believe it is very important to have every study checked by a staff radiologist (or whichever physician will officially "read" the examination) before the patient is dismissed; corralling the individual responsible for this does make the studies a bit longer. The benefits in terms of the diminished need for repeat examination far outweigh the inconvenience.

RECORD KEEPING AND REPORTS

It is important to keep accurate records as to what studies have been performed and when they were done. This will enable you to retrieve studies easily for review and communicate findings quickly to referring physicians. Because most B-scan ultrasonography is carried out in the radiology department, our discussion will be most applicable to such an operation. In the broadest sense, however, the same principles apply no matter where the scanning is done, be it in a radiology department or an obstetrical office.

An index should be kept, listed alphabetically by patients' last names, of all patients examined; each examination should be entered with the type and the date of the study done (Fig. 4–2). In most X-ray departments this will be done as a matter of course; but if not, it is a simple matter to set up a file using 3 × 5 inch cards. We do not believe that data beyond patient name, identifying number, and the date and the type of all examinations need be included on the card.

The actual report should be in narrative form, in the simplest and most direct manner possible. It is preferable that the reports be made on the request form and, therefore, include automatically the pertinent historical data as well as all patient and referring physician identification. At the start of our program in ultrasound, we found that reports which included copies of selective scans were an excellent means of advertising, especially when they were accompanied by hand-drawn identification of findings on the scan. As the volume of our work increased, however, this proved to be a great deal of work for the technologist or the technical aide. At the same time, it appeared that the referring physician was not able or willing to use the copied images and was seldom referring to them, preferring to rely on the written text. What is more, the electrostatic copiers (Xerox and IBM are the two we have used) do not display the gray scale of the scans well, so that the copies were reduced to a few shades of gray, and even that depended heavily on the state of adjustment of the copier. Because of this, we are gradually giving up all but the written report. There is benefit, however, from the extra effort from several aspects. As noted above, the staff becomes more readily familiar with the ultrasound image and is less frightened and/or confused by it. In addition, it is often convenient to have the copied scans in reports in the patients' charts to demonstrate findings when the chart alone is available, for example, at the nurses' station or in working conferences. For these reasons we suggest that at the start of any new ultrasound program, thought be given to including copies of pertinent scans in the reports. For the sake of simplicity and promptness, we use forms with check-off items and blanks to be filled in for reporting our obstetrical cases, and this has proven to be a great saving in time. More will be said about this in Chapter 10.

Copies of the reports should be made a

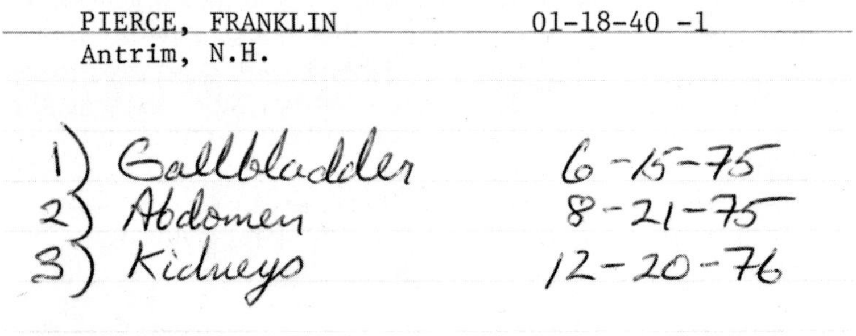

PIERCE, FRANKLIN   01-18-40 -1
Antrim, N.H.

1) Gallbladder   6-15-75
2) Abdomen   8-21-75
3) Kidneys   12-20-76

Figure 4–2. An index listing patients and their examinations is extremely useful. We keep a file on 3 × 5 cards such as this: the cards are arranged in alphabetical order by patient name and contain the type of examination and the date it was performed.

part of the patient's X-ray report file, so that the radiologist or clinician looking to see what studies have been done and what the findings are will have the ultrasound information available. An argument can be made for a separate ultrasound report file; but we believe that if such a separate file is kept, it should be *in addition* to the report filed with the X-ray interpretation. In our hospital, the report to the clinician has been made a part of the X-ray record in the patient's chart. This seems logical in our case, if for no other reason than the fact that we are radiologists. More important, however, ultrasound is an imaging tool and as such provides information closely related to that supplied by radiologic studies. In reviewing the chart, then, it is natural to look in the same place for X-ray and ultrasound findings.

We are of the opinion that the images obtained in an ultrasound examination should be filed with the patient's X-ray films. This keeps all of the radiologic studies together and facilitates review by radiologist and referring physician alike. (Of course, many obstetrical patients will not have an X-ray file packet, and one will have to be made up especially for the ultrasound scan.) The one exception to this method of storing the scans might be in an academic department where rapid access to many ultrasound studies might be needed for the purpose of research. Even here, however, pertinent X-ray films will frequently have to be reviewed; and having the two types of examinations together simplifies this process.

HARD COPY

There are five different types of hard copy available at present to record ultrasound scans. Each has its proponents, its strengths, and its weaknesses. In considering these factors, we will let our own prejudices surface. You will have to weigh many factors in making the decision as to which to use; but, in the main, the three most important are cost, convenience, and quality. The hard copying forms we are going to discuss are Polaroid or instant-developing film (at this writing only film marketed by the Polaroid Corporation is available for scientific work), X-ray film, 70 mm film, heat-sensitive paper, and video tape. We will look at each of these individually.

The first and by far the most widely used recording medium is *Polaroid* Type 107 film, the rapid, self-developing film used for many scientific purposes (Fig. 4–3). Although it is relatively expensive, it is universally available, is an easy-to-use format,

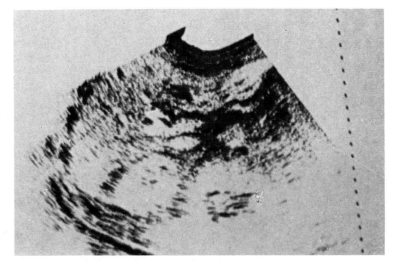

Figure 4–3. Polaroid Type 107 film is the standard hard copy format against which all others are measured. We prefer Type 107 (which is not coated) over Type 107C (the so-called "coaterless" film). If the hard copy monitor is correctly adjusted, Polaroid film can provide an excellent gray scale.

and is generally viewed as the standard against which all other types of hard copy are measured. Polaroid comes in two types useful in scientific work: Type 107, in which coating the picture is recommended, and Type 107C which requires no coating. Type 107 film has a somewhat better latitude than 107C, with distinctly blacker blacks; and it develops in 15 seconds instead of 45 seconds. Development time is not critical, but if the 107C is peeled from its developing material too early, it produces a poor image. By the same token, if the 107C is not peeled relatively soon after development, the image will be lost because it cannot be pulled free. (While the 107 is not so delicate in this regard, it will be destroyed if left unseparated indefinitely, a fact that will become painfully clear to the unfortunate ultrasonographer who unwittingly leaves a study unpeeled for several hours or, even worse, overnight.) In addition, Type 107C Polaroid is slightly more expensive than 107. We prefer Type 107. We have found that the uncoated images do not deteriorate significantly. The main threat to them is scratching; for this reason, if we know we are going to be handling a set of films excessively, we do go to the extra trouble of coating them.

The cost of Polaroid film is high relative to the materials used in other types of hard copying, but there are definite savings in labor and handling. Also, the Polaroid camera itself is inexpensive to buy and is virtually service-free. Unless the volume of work done is very high, the added cost of film is probably of no importance.

The great strength of the self-developing instant film lies in the ready access to images which it provides. The great convenience of having pictures instantly available for study as the patient is being examined, so that findings can be reviewed and confirmed, cannot be overstated. This instant access is extremely important when a relatively inexperienced individual is scanning, and it greatly facilitates review of cases by the physician involved and demonstration of findings in instances where this information is of immediate importance, for example, when amniocentesis or biopsy is being performed.

There is one very important shortcoming of Polaroid film—it is difficult to display the scans to a group using routine X-ray projection apparatus—and in any hospital where there are conferences to attend and house officers to train, this is a serious drawback. It is also cumbersome to keep the Polaroid images sorted for rapid review or display. We have not made use of any of the mounting devices marketed to do this because of their cost and the increased space required for storage. In some laboratories, the pictures are taped together in sequence, using the "permanent" type of Scotch Brand transparent tape. This is quite convenient for demonstration, but it adds significantly to the amount of work required of the scanning and supporting staff. Again, in a small operation and perhaps at the start of an ultrasound program when volume is low and public relations are especially important, taping transverse and then longitudinal scans into separate sequences might be worthwhile.

There are further drawbacks to Polaroid film. Because it requires rather precise exposure control, the camera has to be very carefully set; and the requirement in this regard is somewhat more stringent than with other kinds of film. Also, the latitude of Polaroid film is somewhat narrow. It is certainly adequate, however, for displaying the eight to ten shades of gray of the television monitor. As a practical matter these drawbacks do not interfere seriously in making hard copies with self-developing film.

The next most common types of hard copy are *X-ray* and *70 mm film* (Fig. 4–4, *A* and *B*). As they are essentially similar, we can consider them together. These differ from Polaroid in that they produce a transparent picture on film which can be viewed on an X-ray view box or thrown onto a screen with a standard projector. With the 8 × 10 inch X-ray film format, and to a lesser extent with the 70 mm film as well, multiple images can be put on the same piece of film.

There is a distinct saving in the cost of materials with either X-ray or 70 mm film. The saving is offset, however, by increased cost of film handling (dark-room, personnel, time), as well as in the initial cost of many of the instruments used for making these images. The independent camera systems which use X-ray film and which have a video monitor separate from the

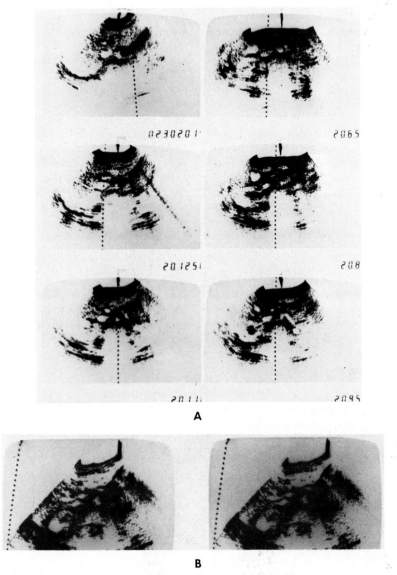

A

B

Figure 4-4. Clear base films, such as X-ray or 70 mm film, have some advantages and disadvantages when compared to Polaroid film. Both X-ray film (*A*) and 70 mm film (*B*) provide excellent images.

scanner (Dunn or Matrix, for example) are expensive and require service in addition to the capital costs. It is possible, however, to obtain 70 mm or X-ray film pictures with adaptors fitted to the back of the camera attached to the scanner's video screen. These are inexpensive; and because they are manually operated, they are generally reliable. (Such camera backs lack the versatility of the independent systems in that they do not offer variable formats.) Both X-ray and 70 mm films have greater latitude than the Polaroid; and, therefore, exposure control is not as critical. They also have a greater density range than reflected light prints. For these reasons, the images are often much more pleasing to view. More importantly, however, they lend themselves admirably to display in conferences and lectures and are much easier to use in a teaching setting. They can also be readily copied.

In the case of X-ray or 70 mm film, the trade-off is with convenience. The technologist must have access to a means of developing the film, and it is not possible to lay out the scans as they are made to keep track of what has been seen. This inability to check previous scans easily has been mentioned above and is referred to once again because of its great importance. In addition, however, it is hard to edit the scans with either 70 mm or X-ray films; that is, it is difficult to put the studies in proper order. Suppose a sequence of transverse scans is made at 10, 11, and 12 centimeters above the iliac crest and later it is found that ones at 10.5, 11.5, and 12.5 centimeters would also be helpful. With either the 70 mm or the X-ray film format, sequencing after the images are made and recorded is awkward. In the case of 70 mm film there is the added disadvantage that the film cassettes are often difficult to load and unload. This puts an added burden on the already busy ultrasound technologist.

Another type of hard copy imaging involves the use of *heat-sensitive paper* (Fig. 4–5). The original copiers could reproduce only bi-stable images and were suitable only for bi-stable scanning. The latest models, however, are reputed to make satisfactory images in gray scale. The output is a sheet of opaque paper, 8 × 10 inches in dimension, and it is produced in seconds without having to be processed in a separate developer. The images are somewhat less satisfactory than Polaroid in terms of quality, and they are cumbersome to handle because of their size. In addition, the

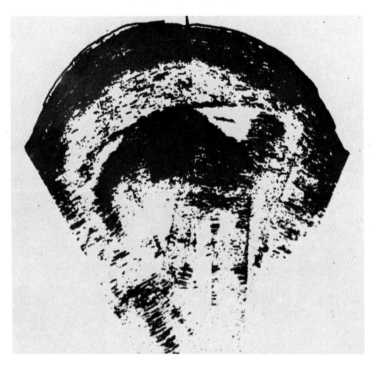

Figure 4–5. Heat-sensitive paper has enjoyed some popularity as a hard copy medium for bi-stable scans. The large size and poor gray rendition have limited its use in gray-scale scanning, however.

copying apparatus is expensive and requires frequent servicing. Recording with heat-sensitive paper does have the convenience of speed, ease of operation, and inexpensive materials. Overall, in our opinion this format does not seem to offer enough advantags to supplant other hard copy systems.

Finally, we should say a word regarding *video tape.* It is easy to record ultrasound scans on video tape if you are using gray scale. It does not require a fancy video-recorder; the least expensive one will do, and anyone acquainted with such electronic gear can hook it up, usually with little or no modification of the ultrasound scanner. How would this be of any use? Well, it would allow the technologist to scan almost at random and later edit the scans, recording only those which are pertinent. Then, if an X-ray film recorder were used, the scans could be recorded in proper sequence. This is really a luxury, probably appropriate only in a big ultrasound lab; but it does add an element of flexibility. Certainly, video tape has no place as the sole recording medium; it is simply too cumbersome for the retrieval of data. On the other hand, when a real time scanner is used, because of the nature of the scanning instrument video tape is essential.

Now, what format do we prefer? We find it hard to give up Polaroid because of its speed and great convenience. Because we find ourselves increasingly in need of demonstrating our findings to others in large groups, we are using the X-ray film format more and more. We use a relatively inexpensive commercial adaptor which fits on the back of the camera in place of the standard Polaroid back. This performs the same function as a very expensive automatic camera, although it is fixed in its format and is somewhat less convenient to use. For most laboratories, however, we see no reason to go beyond Polaroid.

Any scanning system should have a means of recording identification data on the scan image. Many scanners have character generators built in, and this option makes identification very easy. Typing patient identification data, the date, and even the position of the scan is simply and rapidly done. If your scanner does not have such a device, you can rather easily take apart a cheap hand calculator and install its read-out over the lower portion of the TV screen so that it is photographed with the scan image. With this device at least the patient's identification number can be recorded on each scan image.

Well, now that your lab is set up, we can move on to more exciting things and begin to take a look at the scan itself.

Chapter 5

ARTIFACTS

Before we discuss actual scanning procedures we need to examine the problem of artifact production in some detail because it is hard to overestimate the importance of artifacts in day-to-day scanning. Between one third and one half of the dots which appear on the image are artifacts (in some scanning situations this amount may be closer to 90 per cent). If we parceled out words on this basis, we would devote six chapters to artifacts, instead of only one! Although there has been some discussion of artifacts in the literature and in other texts, we feel that the subject has been shortchanged. It is unsettling to see case after case in which artifacts are mislabeled as real structures and whole discussions and clinical signs developed — all concerning echoes which are not real. At the World Congress of Ultrasound held in San Francisco in August, 1976, there were many papers presented in which artifacts were discussed as if they were real echoes. (One particularly memorable presentation discussed a new ultrasonic sign — unfortunately the "echoes" the author was describing were all artifacts!) Since artifacts are so prevalent and since they occur in all types of examinations, it is important to understand where they come from, what they look like, and how to avoid them or diminish their impact before we take up individual scanning situations.

When we say that as many as half of the echoes in the picture are artifacts you may be skeptical; however, the same situation holds in much of radiology. Scattered radiation is, in effect, an artifact on an X-ray film. An abdominal X-ray film, even with a grid, not infrequently contains 50 per cent scattered radiation; a tomogram of the kidneys contains a much higher percentage. The fact that so much of the image is artifactual radiation does not diminish the value of the X-ray film; the radiologist learns to recognize and ignore the scattered radiation and concentrate on what is real. (Of course, steps are taken to reduce scatter as much as possible with grids, air gaps, high KV and the like.) Similarly, in ultrasound, the presence of artifacts need not ruin an image as long as we recognize the artifacts for what they are and take steps to avoid them as much as possible.

TYPES OF ARTIFACTS

Perhaps we should have a more precise definition of "artifact" before we proceed further. The standard dictionary definition is "something made by skilled human hands" — thus the "artifacts" of ancient Greece are things which were made by skilled hands. Clearly, this is not the type of artifact with which we are concerned (truly skilled hands should be able to avoid ultrasound artifacts). The accepted medical definition is more appropriate — "anything that is caused by the technique used and is not a natural occurrence." This is still a somewhat awkward description. We shall consider an **artifact** as any dot which appears in the ultrasound image which does not correspond to a real echo in the patient. Although artifacts can arise from many sources, there are only three causes of most artifacts encountered in clinical scanning: (1) electronic noise or interferences, (2) signal processing artifacts, and (3) reverberations.

Electronic noise can take many forms. In any electronic device (such as a transistor, capacitor, inductor, or rectifier) electrons move about randomly. When a signal is applied to such a device the electrons tend to move in a specified pattern; however, there is always some randomness to this movement and, at any given instant in time, there may be some electrons moving in the wrong direction. This random movement gives rise to very tiny but real electric voltages which are not part of the main signal. These tiny signals are referred to as "electronic noise." This definition was formulated in the early days of radio when the tiny signals from the random electron movement came out as background noise on the loudspeaker. (The same noise still exists. If you set your radio dial in between stations, there will be a familiar buzzing sound which is the electronic noise in the radio. Higher quality radios have better circuitry and less noise, but even the most expensive FM receivers still have a small background noise level.)

Electronic noise does not have to appear as sound: it will appear in the same form as the output of the system. Thus, a slight flickering of a fluorescent light can represent noise in its power supply circuit. After the late-night movie, a prayer, and The Star-Spangled Banner (complete with jet planes and rockets) have been run and your favorite TV station signs off for the night there will be nothing but "snow" on your TV set; this "snow" is made up, in part, by electronic noise in the TV. Similarly, the background electronic noise in an ultrasound scanner can produce tiny dots in the image. The signals producing the noise are very small compared to the signals from the echoes and will produce only very light gray dots on the screen. These signals are usually so small that they appear only when the amplifier sensitivity is set at a very high level. If the sounder or scan converter is out of adjustment, however, the noise may become more prominent and intrude on an image produced at normal gain. The best way to avoid this type of artifact is to have the scanner properly "tuned up," because in a well-tuned scanner the background noise levels are too small to interfere with the picture.

Interference from outside high-frequency signals is another form of electronic noise artifact. We have probably all had the experience of watching a TV picture go berserk at a critical moment because an airplane flew overhead or some hot-rodder drove by in a car without ignition suppression. The TV picked up the outside signal and superimposed it on the real signal. This same phenomenon can occur with an ultrasound scanner. High-frequency radio transmission from a nearby source can generate a snowstorm of tiny echoes on the screen. (An even more common problem in a hospital setting is interference from the "Bovie," the electrocautery device frequently used in operating rooms. We have experienced considerable artifact production on bi-stable scans when the Bovie was in use, but have not noticed this to be a major problem with gray scale.)

Artifacts may be introduced into the ultrasound picture by the design of the signal processing. For instance, in bi-stable scanners there is a very common artifact known as the "loud echo artifact." This artifact arises when leading edge display is used. In order to convert the spikes in the A-mode to the dots required for B-mode, the sounder must have some method of recognizing when one echo stops and another echo starts. This is usually done by recognizing a "leading edge" — a departure of the electric signal from the baseline. Every time the signal leaves the zero level a B-mode dot is generated. When the echoes are small and the resulting electric signals small, there is no problem. When a very loud echo is received, however, the electric signal may be so large that it cannot return to baseline before the next signal is received. Because the subsequent echo signal did not start at baseline, it is not recognized by the scanner and no B-mode dot is generated. The result is that there is a blind area immediately following loud echoes. No B-mode dots can be generated in this area and on the picture it appears echoless even though echoes may be present. Figure 5–1 illustrates a loud echo artifact. If a loud echo artifact is suspected, the ultrasonographer should switch to A-mode where the true nature of the echoes will be apparent. Another option is to stay in B-mode and turn *down* the gain. This seemingly paradoxical adjustment will decrease all echo signals and enable the "loud echo" signal to return to baseline, thereby giving the following signals a chance to be recorded.

Loud echo artifacts are not a problem in gray scale scanners; however, other forms of signal processing may cause image distortion in these machines. As we saw in Chapter 3, the type of signal processing employed distorts the final image. Most of these modifications result in overall improvement of the picture; but it must be appreciated that the cost of this is loss of some information. If the scanner "smooths"

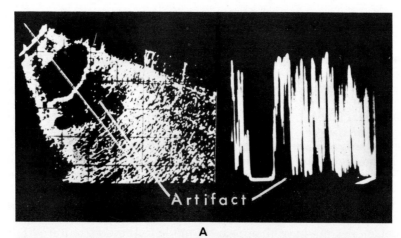

A

B

Figure 5–1. The "loud echo" artifact is an electronic artifact seen in bi-stable scanners when the gain is set too high. A B-mode dot is generated every time the A-mode tracing departs from baseline; if the gain is so high that a "loud echo" cannot return to baseline before the next echo is received, the second echo will not be recorded on the B-mode display.

A, A B-mode scan through a dilated gallbladder and the A-mode tracing corresponding to the line drawn on the scan. The back wall of the gallbladder gives such a loud echo that the A-mode tracing does not return to baseline for several microseconds: during this period no new B-mode dots can be generated and there is an artifactual echoless area behind the gallbladder.

B, The same scan with the gain reduced so that the A-mode echoes return to baseline. The "echoless" area behind the gallbladder has filled in, confirming that it was an artifact.

the picture by broadening the echoes so they emerge smoothly, some small echoes may be obscured and the edges of the organs will become less distinct. A scanner which stresses edge enhancement may give well-delineated margins but a very "grainy" picture in which it may be difficult to appreciate the overall anatomy. Too much edge enhancement may promote otherwise innocuous electronic noise to the status of echo. There is nothing that the ultrasonographer can do about these signal processing artifacts except acknowledge their existence. Fortunately, they do not seem to have a significant adverse effect on the

diagnostic quality of the ultrasound image.

The same thing cannot be said for reverberation artifacts — these are a real bugaboo in B-mode scanning, so we will look at them in detail.

ORIGIN OF REVERBERATION ARTIFACTS

Up until now we have been assuming that the ultrasound beam makes a straightforward trip to an interface and back to the transducer, where it generates a signal. We have not considered the fate of the pulse once it has hit the crystal. Some of it is absorbed by the crystal and the damping material in the transducer, but a significant portion is reflected back into the patient. After all, the transducer–soft tissue interface constitutes a gigantic acoustic impedance mismatch which makes it a very effective ultrasonic reflector. So our pulse bounces off the transducer and makes a second trip through the patient to the interface, where another echo is produced which returns to the transducer. At the transducer the same thing happens: a signal is generated and what is left of the beam is reflected back into the patient for a third trip. (Of course, the pulse is much weaker now, having been attenuated by two trips through the patient.) This process of the pulse bouncing back and forth between two interfaces is known as **reverberation**; and it will continue until the pulse is totally exhausted by attenuation. (Our friend who is measuring the canyon sometimes experiences reverberation if he is standing at the bottom of it when he shouts. The canyon wall behind him will act as the second interface and his shouted "Hello" keeps bounding back and forth— "HELLO"... hello-hello-hello-hello. . . .)

It is easy to see how reverberation will produce artifacts in our image. Each time the reverberating pulse strikes the crystal it generates a signal. The sounder has no way of knowing that the signal arose from reverberation; all it knows is that the signal was received in twice the time as the first signal (or three times or four times, depending on how long the reverberation persists). The sounder records the signals generated by the reverberating pulse just as if they were real echoes and places each at the distance corresponding to the time it was received. Figure 5–2 illustrates a reverberating pulse and shows how the sounder would record this pulse in A- and B-mode. There are several things to notice about the reverberation and its artifacts. (1) Only the initial spike (or dot in B-mode) is real; it corresponds to the original echo from the interface. (2) The spikes from each of the reverberations are recorded in multiples of the distance of the interface; that is, the first artifactual spike will be twice as far from the transducer as the real echo, the second artifact will be three times this distance, and so forth. It is obvious why this occurs: the first reverberation had to make two trips to

the interface and back and thus took twice as long to be received; the next reverberation had to make three trips, etc. (3) Each artifact spike is smaller than the previous one because the reverberating pulse is continually being attenuated by the tissue. In B-mode gray scale this would manifest as each dot being a lighter shade of gray than its predecessor.

If we examine Figure 5–2, *B* we will be able to recognize conditions in which reverberation artifacts will be severe. First, the louder the echo, the more likely it is to produce reverberations. Unless the echo is strong it will not have enough amplitude to make the return journey to the interface without being completely attenuated. Echoes which arise from soft tissue–bone interfaces (such as ribs) or soft tissue–air interfaces (such as bowel gas) are loud enough to generate a significant number of reverberation artifacts. In general, echoes arising from soft tissue interfaces do not have sufficient amplitude to set up reverberations; however, this is not invariably true. If the interface is a large, specular reflector which is located at right angles to the sound beam and is fairly close to the transducer so that there is little attenuation, reverberation artifacts can occur. The fascial planes of the anterior abdominal wall fulfill these criteria and frequently produce linear artifacts in the underlying tissue (Fig. 5–3).

Second, we can see that more reverberations will be produced at high gain than at low gain. Increasing the gain gives all echoes more amplitude and means that more reverberations will survive tissue attenuation to cause artifacts. When using a bi-stable scanner it is possible for much of the scan to keep the gain low enough so that few reverberations occur. Gray scale scanning is done at very high gain, however, and this makes reverberation an especially troublesome problem.

Finally, the nearer an interface is located to the transducer, the more likely it is to cause reverberation artifacts. This is partly because there is greater attenuation of the echo from distant interfaces and hence the pulse is more likely to die out before it can reverberate. An even more important factor is the size of the image, however. Remember that the first artifact occurs at *twice* the distance the interface actually is from the transducer. If the interface is at 3

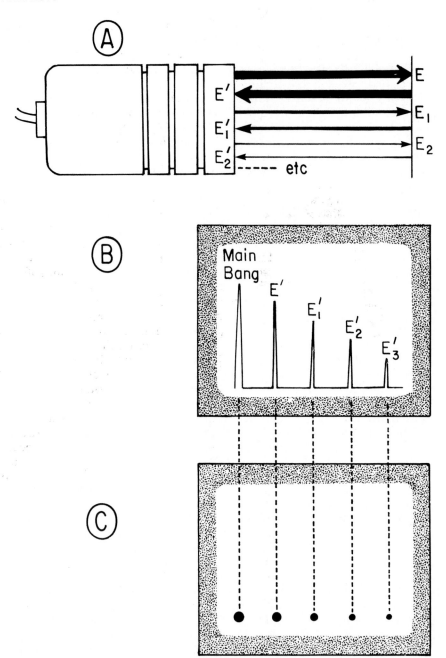

Figure 5–2. The reverberations of an echo between the transducer and an interface cause artifacts.

A, The initial pulse (*large arrow*) leaves the transducer and travels to an interface where echo, E, is produced. When the echo returns to the transducer it generates an electric signal, E'. However, the echo is reflected back into the tissue and makes a second trip to the interface (*arrow*) where another echo, E_1, is produced. When this echo returns to the transducer, it generates a second electric signal, E'_1, and is again reflected into the tissue (*small arrow*), where an additional echo, E_2, and signal, E'_2, are produced. This procedure continues until the pulse is exhausted by attenuation.

B, The A-mode presentation of the reverberation process shows one real echo signal, E', and several artifactual signals, E'_1 to E'_3. Notice that each of the artifacts occurs at a multiple of the distance to the real echo, that is, the distance from the main bang to spike E' is the same as the distance from E' to E'_1, or from E'_1 to E'_2, or E'_2 to E'_3. Because of attenuation, each succeeding spike is of smaller amplitude, and eventually the signals die out.

C, In B-mode the reverberations present as a series of dots of decreasing brightness. Only the first dot corresponds to a real echo in the patient; the others are all artifacts.

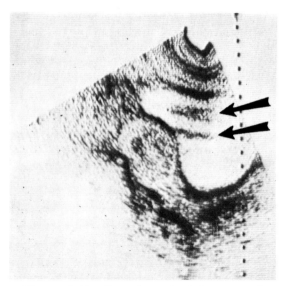

Figure 5-3. Reverberations between the body wall and the transducer face produce artifacts. In this longitudinal scan of a normal pelvis (notice the IUD in the uterus) there are two prominent linear artifacts in the upper portion of the bladder (*arrows*). It is easy to see the real echo interfaces which gave rise to these artifacts in the overlying soft tissue.

centimeters, the first artifact will occur at 6 centimeters. (Where will the second and third artifacts occur?) This artifact which occurs at 6 centimeters will be superimposed on the real image. Now suppose that an interface at 7 centimeters gives rise to an artifact; this artifact will occur at 14 centimeters and, most of the time, will fall outside of the useful image (most B-scans are limited to a depth of 10 to 20 centimeters as there are very few transducer-TCG combinations which are capable of deeper penetration). As long as the artifacts are projected beyond the useful image they create no problem. (In some experimental scanning set-ups the patient is scanned through a water bath. One advantage of this arrangement is that the first echo does not occur until 10 to 12 centimeters and hence the first artifact occurs at 20 to 24 centimeters and is projected beyond the image. This is, in many ways, analogous to using an air gap to decrease scattered radiation in X-rays.)

In summary, then, reverberation artifacts are most serious in the near field (that is, within 5 centimeters of the transducer), when scanning at high gain, over loud echo interfaces.

COMMON REVERBERATION ARTIFACTS

We have already mentioned one situation where these artifacts are common — the fascial planes of the abdominal wall. Figures 5-3 and 5-4 show examples of this problem. We are all familiar with the over-knowledgeable wise guy in a hospital — the one who thinks he is an expert in every field and who would never deign to ask a question or admit he did not know something. We have found that these individu-

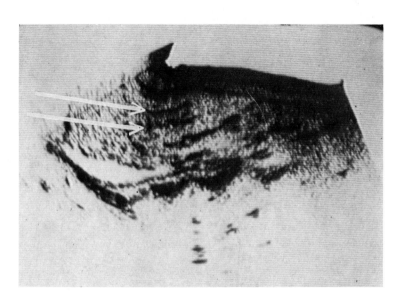

Figure 5-4. Reverberation artifacts are harder to recognize when they are projected onto normal echo-producing areas. In this longitudinal scan through the right lobe of the liver there are two linear reverberation artifacts from the overlying body wall (*white arrows*) superimposed on the normal liver echoes.

als are usually stumped when asked to explain the "echoes" in the upper part of the bladder, as shown in Figure 5–3. They mumble something about "tumor" or "infection" but almost never consider that these "echoes" could not be real. In fact, these "echoes" are *not* real, they are merely reverberation artifacts from the fascial planes of the abdominal wall.

(*Homework time:* The full urinary bladder is an excellent way to visualize the concept of reverberation artifacts. We know that the bladder does not produce any real echoes—it contains no interfaces—and hence, any "echoes" which appear in its upper portion are artifacts. Drink three beers and then go scan your bladder. Be sure to keep the transducer over the bladder—we will explain why in a moment—and make a series of scans; start at low gain and slowly increase the gain as you scan. The low-gain pictures should have no "echoes" within the bladder but as the gain is increased, reverberation artifacts will begin to appear. These will first be in the very top of the bladder; as the gain is progressively increased they will penetrate deeper and deeper until they obscure the entire bladder, even its back wall. Now move the transducer up to your umbilicus and try to scan the bladder from

this position by angling the transducer toward your pelvis. Can you outline the bladder? Can you even find the bladder? Why are the images of the bladder so poor when it is scanned from the umbilicus? We will see in a minute.)

It is not a difficult matter to recognize reverberation artifacts in the bladder; after all, there are no real echoes there. Things are not so obvious when the scan is performed over soft tissue where there are real echoes as well as the artifacts. Figure 5–4 shows the artifacts from the abdominal wall projected into the liver. Notice that they have the same general appearance as they did when projected in the bladder; however, they are more difficult to recognize because of the real echoes originating from liver tissue in the same area.

Soft tissue–bone interfaces generate many artifacts. In abdominal and pelvic scanning this usually occurs when the sound beam is passed through a rib. Figure 5–5 shows an artifact from a rib projected into an enlarged spleen. The xiphoid process, when heavily calcified, gives rise to artifacts in the left lobe of the liver, as illustrated in Figure 5–6.

The champion artifact producer is the soft tissue–air interface. The bowel, from stomach to rectum, is a source of these in-

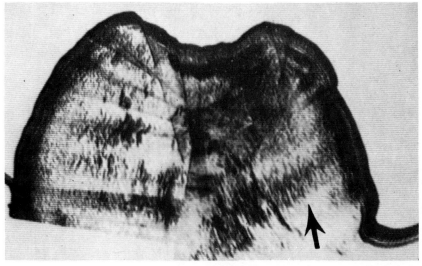

Figure 5–5. Ribs give rise to very strong reverberation artifacts. In this transverse abdominal scan of a patient with an enlarged spleen there is a large rib artifact traversing the spleen (*arrow*). Notice similar artifacts in the liver from other ribs. It is important to recognize that the *dots*, not the *white spaces*, are the artifacts.

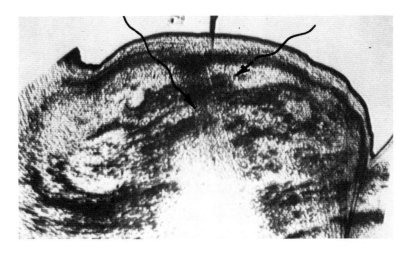

Figure 5–6. The calcified xiphoid process can generate reverberation artifacts which are projected onto the left lobe of the liver and central pancreas. This is a high transverse scan of a normal abdomen. When the transducer was moved over the xiphoid process, artifacts (*wiggly black arrows*) were produced in the underlying structures.

terfaces and causes the majority of artifacts which plague the abdominal and pelvic scan. There is always gas in the stomach and colon and usually some in the small intestine as well: thus, when the sound beam is passed through bowel, the potential for artifact production is high.

Figure 5–7 shows reverberation artifacts from gas in the hepatic flexure of the colon. Back in Chapter 1 we discovered that the acoustic impedance mismatch between gas and soft tissue was so great that over 99 per cent of the sound beam was reflected; this

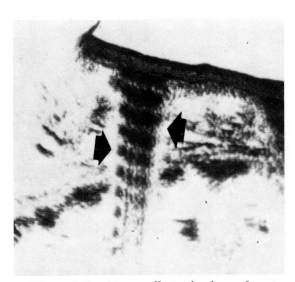

Figure 5–7. Air, usually in the form of gas in the bowel, produces dramatic reverberation artifacts. This longitudinal scan through the right lobe of the liver shows the steplike artifacts produced by air in the hepatic flexure of the colon (*short arrows*).

explains why gas produces so many artifacts — it is an excellent reflector and can bounce a large percentage of the beam back to the transducer. Even if the amount of gas is small — only a few bubbles, for instance — there will be many artifacts produced. Figure 5–8 shows bowel gas artifacts projected into the aorta. This is a normal aorta which does not give rise to internal echoes at normal gain settings. The "echoes" which we see in the aorta are actually artifacts produced by small amounts of gas in the overlying small bowel.

Of course large amounts of gas make large artifacts. Figure 5–9 shows an extremely common bowel gas artifact arising from gas in the stomach. Most people have a moderate amount of air in the stomach; and when they lie supine (the position for most abdominal scanning), this air rises to the gastric antrum, just underneath the left lobe of the liver. It has two effects: first, since it reflects 99 per cent of the sound beam, it totally obscures the underlying tissue (no matter how high the gain is turned there is no way to penetrate gas); and, second, it generates large showers of echoes which are projected into the underlying tissue. It is very important that the ultrasonographer understand these two points (and very distressing that apparently many people scanning today do not). Therefore, please indulge us while we beat this horse to death.

When the sound beam encounters bowel gas, it is totally blocked; there is no way to "blast" through it by turning up the gain; and, consequently, there is no way to gen-

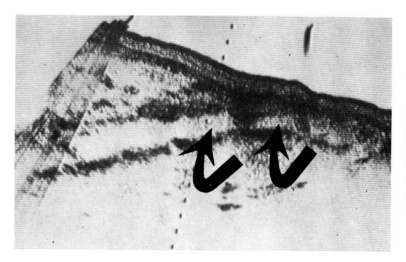

Figure 5–8. Subtle reverberation artifacts can be very difficult to recognize. In this longitudinal scan through the aorta there are several "clouds" of small echoes in the lumen of the lower aorta (*curved arrows*). These are not real echoes; they are artifacts from small amounts of gas in the overlying bowel.

erate echoes from underlying structures. Any "echoes" which appear under bowel gas are artifacts, no matter what the gain setting or how dark the "echoes." Of course, at low gain there are fewer artifacts than at high gain; this probably accounts for the common misconception that increasing the gain blasts the sound beam through the gas.

SUBTLE ARTIFACTS

Artifacts are insidious things and can lead the unwary ultrasonographer astray in many ways. We have already seen how they clutter up the picture and cause confusion with real echoes, but this is only part of the problem.

Figure 5–10 illustrates how they can totally obscure organ boundaries and real echoes. Figure 5–10, *A* is a longitudinal scan through the right lobe of the liver; the transducer was always kept over the liver and the sound beam not allowed to pass through bowel. The image of the liver is satisfactory. Figure 5–10, *B* is the same scan as in 5–10, *A* except that the transducer was moved past the liver and onto bowel. When the sound beam passed through bowel gas, it generated artifacts; and, when the transducer was aimed back toward the

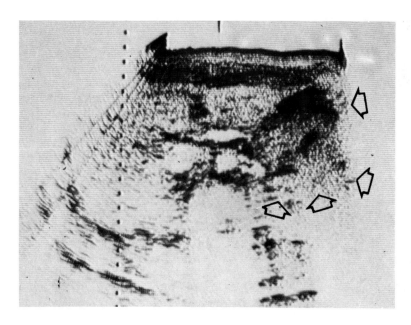

Figure 5–9. The left upper quadrant of the abdomen is frequently obscured by bowel gas artifacts. This transverse scan of a normal upper abdomen shows a typical appearance of the artifacts which arise from air in the stomach or splenic flexure of the colon (*open arrows*). No matter how little air is in the stomach, when the patient is supine this air rises to the gastric antrum where it is in an excellent position to cause artifacts.

A

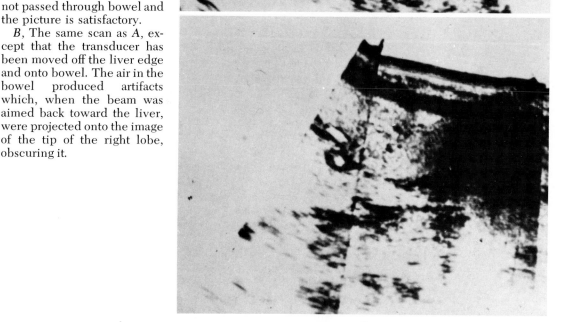

B

Figure 5-10. If the sound beam is allowed to pass through bowel or rib, the artifacts produced may obscure an otherwise useful image.

A, A longitudinal scan through the right lobe of the liver: the sound beam has not passed through bowel and the picture is satisfactory.

B, The same scan as *A,* except that the transducer has been moved off the liver edge and onto bowel. The air in the bowel produced artifacts which, when the beam was aimed back toward the liver, were projected onto the image of the tip of the right lobe, obscuring it.

liver, these artifacts were projected into the liver, obscuring the tip of the right lobe.

Figure 5-11 shows this same phenomenon arising from a rib. Figure 5-11, *A* is a longitudinal scan of the kidney; the transducer was kept over the soft tissue and the sound beam not allowed to pass through a rib. The upper pole is seen well. Figure 5-11, *B* is the same scan except that the transducer was scanned over the twelfth rib. The rib produced artifacts which were projected into the kidney, obscuring its upper pole.

These two cases illustrate artifact problems which, while serious, are fairly easy to recognize. When there are several disconnected artifacts, they may be more difficult to appreciate, however. Consider the scans of the liver shown in Figure 5-12. These scans were performed at the same level, at the same time, in the same patient; the only difference was technique. Figure 5-12, *A* was obtained with a poor scanning technique: the transducer was scanned over the entire right chest wall *including the ribs.* Every time the sound beam passed through a rib a string of artifacts was produced and projected into the liver. Several strings of artifacts, each corresponding to a different rib, are apparent in the image. The overall picture of the liver is heterogeneous and might be mistaken for a liver full

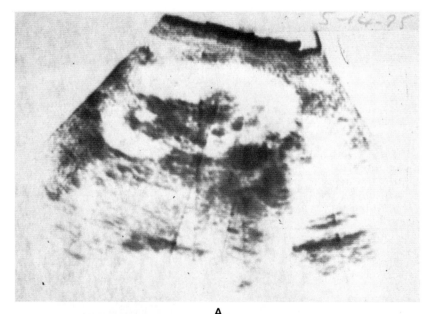

A

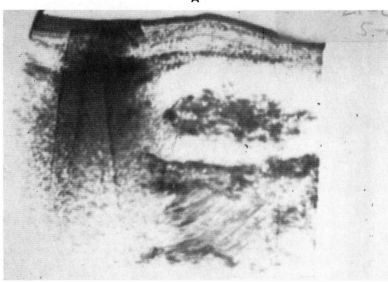

B

Figure 5–11. Passing the sound beam through a rib can generate artifacts which confuse underlying anatomy.

A, A longitudinal scan of the kidney: the transducer was not moved over rib and the upper pole of the kidney is nicely defined.

B, The same scan as *A*, except that the transducer has been moved over the twelfth rib: the resulting artifacts have obscured the upper pole of the kidney.

of metastases. Figure 5–12, *B* was obtained using proper scanning technique and shows that the liver is normal. The transducer was kept over the soft tissues and sectored through the liver; at no time was the beam passed through ribs or bowel. (There are more shortcomings to the scanning technique of Figure 5–12, *A* than simply artifact production: transducer-skin contact is poor between ribs and this results in excessive attenuation of echoes; also the sound beam is scanned across some deeper echoes more than one time. We will discuss scanning technique in detail in Chapter 6.)

Isolated artifactual echoes can be mis-

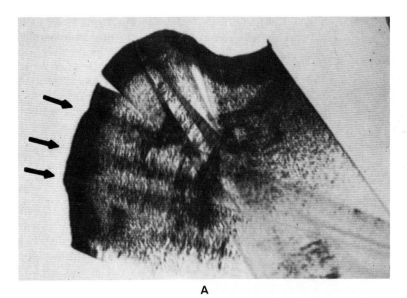

A

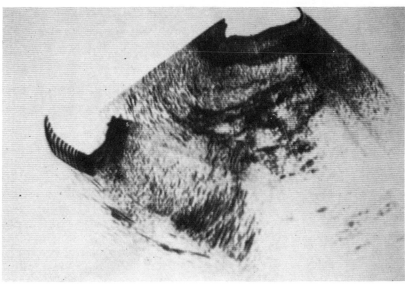

B

Figure 5–12. The sound beam must not pass through a rib when scanning the liver.

A, A transverse scan of a normal liver: the transducer was moved across the entire body wall, including ribs. Each time the sound beam traversed a rib an artifact was produced in the liver (*arrows*); this heterogeneous echo pattern could be misinterpreted as liver disease.

B, The same scan of the same liver as in A, except that the sound beam was not allowed to pass through a rib: the true nature of the parenchyma is now apparent and the liver is normal.

taken for organ or mass boundaries and can lead to erroneous diagnoses. Figure 5–13 illustrates such a case. This patient had had lung cancer in the past and was sent for ultrasound examination because of a small, palpable mass just under the left rib cage. Figure 5–13, A shows the ultrasound scan at the level of this palpable mass. Because of poor technique the sound beam was allowed to pass through an adjacent rib, causing an artifact. This was not recognized as a rib artifact by the ultrasonographer and was interpreted instead as the back wall of the mass. The spleen was identified on other sections and was not located in this region: therefore, the ultrasonographer

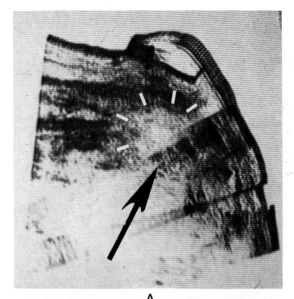

A

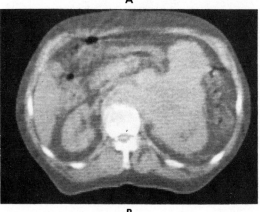

B

Figure 5–13. Artifacts can create artificial boundaries.

A, A technically poor transverse scan of the left upper abdomen; there is a rib artifact (*black arrow*) which was misinterpreted as the posterior wall of the mass outlined by the small white marks. Because of this the ultrasound diagnosis was "small, resectable tumor."

B, A CT scan of the same area shows the true extent of the mass: it is quite large, involving the left kidney and retroperitoneum, and surgery is not indicated.

came to the conclusion that the palpable mass was quite small and confined to the area immediately underneath the rib cage where it could be easily removed.

If the rib artifact had been recognized for what it was (or better yet, if it had never occurred), the ultrasonographer would have seen that the mass was actually much larger and involved most of the left upper abdomen. Figure 5–13, *B* is a CT scan of the same area and shows the true size of the mass; it is clear that surgery would have been inappropriate for the patient. (*Humility department,* or, "Never get cocky, it can happen to you": Despite the fact that we have been lecturing and warning about this problem for several years, one of us (RJB) was the errant ultrasonographer in this case. Among the lessons to be learned is that there is no substitute for meticulous scanning technique; a technically poor scan is an invitation to misdiagnosis.)

INTERNAL REVERBERATION ARTIFACTS

We have been discussing reverberation artifacts which arise from the sound beam's being reflected off the transducer face; although these reverberations are by far the most troublesome in clinical scanning, they are not the only type of reverberation artifact which occurs. As the echo returns to the transducer it encounters many interfaces and at each there is the potential for a portion of the echo to be reflected back into the patient. Figure 5–14 illustrates how internal reverberations arise. In this schematized diagram we follow a single pulse on its journey to a cyst and back. The pulse reaches the front wall of the cyst and an echo is produced, which returns to the transducer. The pulse continues on to the back wall of the cyst where another echo is

Figure 5–14. The reverberation of an echo between two internal interfaces can produce artifacts, as illustrated in lines 1 to 6. Line 1 shows a pulse passing through an interface, A, and producing echo A'. In line 2 the pulse crosses interface B, producing echo B'. (Interfaces A and B can be thought of as the front and back walls of a cyst.) When the echo B' recrosses interface A (line 3) some of it will be reflected back into the cyst. When this reflected portion encounters interface B, a second echo, B'$_1$, is produced (line 4). Line 5 shows that as this echo B'$_1$ crosses interface A again a small portion will be reflected. In line 6 echo B'$_1$ has returned to the transducer while the reflected portion is again encountering the back wall of the cyst, producing another echo, B'$_2$.

The right side of each line shows the A-mode oscilloscope tracing of these echoes. A' and B' are, of course, the true echoes from interfaces A and B; but B'$_1$ (and B'$_2$, B'$_3$, etc.) are artifacts.

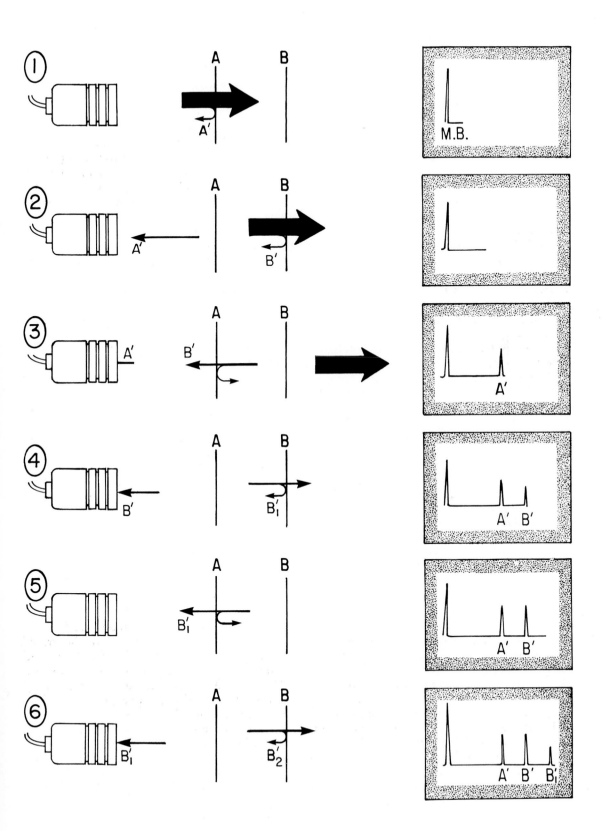

Figure 5-14. See opposite page for legend.

produced. The pulse then continues on through the patient, but we will forget about it and now follow the progress of the echo produced at the back wall of the cyst. This echo starts its return journey to the transducer, but when it reaches the front wall of the cyst, a small portion of it is reflected back into the cyst. (Remember that an interface reflects sound no matter which direction the beam is traveling when it crosses it.) The portion of our echo which was not reflected back into the cyst continues on to the transducer. The reflected portion returns to the back wall of the cyst where it is once again bounced back toward the transducer. When the reflected portion arrives at the transducer, it will produce a signal which, since it was delayed on its return by the "extra" journey in the cyst, will not be recorded in the proper position, but will be located deeper in the image.

An alternative method of conceptualizing internal reverberations is to understand that small portions of echoes get delayed on their return trip to the transducer. The delays are caused by internal reflections (or reverberations) from interfaces that the echoes cross on their return trip. Any echo which is delayed in its return journey will produce an artifact, since the sounder always assumes that the echo made a direct trip to the interface and back and places the dot in the image in a position which is equivalent to a direct trip.

Because the amount of delay depends on the number of reverberations the echo undergoes before it finally returns to the transducer, and because this number is extremely variable, it is not possible to predict where the artifacts will be projected into the image (unlike reverberations from the transducer face where the artifacts are projected at multiples of the original distance). It is, therefore, extremely difficult to recognize the artifacts produced by internal reverberations (for all practical purposes they are impossible to distinguish from real echoes). Fortunately for clinical ultrasonography, the interfaces in the body are not nearly as good reflectors as the transducer face so the percentage of echoes which survive attenuation to produce internal reverberation artifacts is small and rarely compromises the diagnostic useful-ness of the image. Only gas and bone give rise to significant numbers of internal reverberation artifacts.

THE ACOUSTIC WINDOW

After this dissertation on the plague of artifacts which complicate the ultrasound image you may be tempted to give up ultrasound and take up ditch-digging or some other more straightforward field. Do not despair; all is not lost. It is true that artifacts are ever present in ultrasound scanning but, as we said earlier, once the ultrasonographer accepts that fact, learns to recognize the artifacts, and takes steps to avoid them, he will be able to produce diagnostically useful images in the majority of patients.

We have already learned how to recognize many of these villains; it is now time to turn our attention to avoiding them. We have mentioned most of the things which can be done in this regard. First, we must always *scan at the lowest gain which is compatible with a good image.* Once artifacts are encountered it does no good to increase the gain to try to "see" through them. (We will discuss how to set the gain controls in Chapter 6.) In this regard it is often useful to use low frequency transducers which can reach deeper structures with less gain than higher frequency transducers.

Next, we can *avoid scanning in situations or areas which are prone to produce artifacts.* This is the most important way to avoid artifacts. The ultrasound beam should never be allowed to pass through a rib or gas-bearing bowel if this can be avoided, and most of the time it can. When the upper abdomen is scanned, the transducer should be kept over the liver and sectored throughout the region of interest. The transducer should never be scanned across ribs; if the deeper portions of the right lobe of the liver are not visible from the anterior abdominal wall, the transducer should be placed *between* ribs and another sector scan performed. When scanning the pelvis, it is absolutely imperative that the patient have a full bladder. The bladder lifts the bowel out of the pelvis and permits the sound beam to reach the pelvic organs without having to traverse artifact-producing bowel gas. In scanning the kidneys the patient is turned prone so that the sound can reach the kidneys via the muscles of the back rather than through the bowel (of course we must be careful not to scan over the twelfth rib).

This process of avoiding bowel and bone is sometimes referred to as scanning through an **acoustic window.** We think this is a very good description of an important concept: in ultrasound scanning there are "acoustic walls" and "acoustic windows"; the sound beam can "see" through the windows but not the walls. Bone and bowel (with its ever-present gas) are the walls; passing the beam through them is very likely to produce artifacts and render the image less useful. Soft tissue is the window; scanning through soft tissue gives the most reliable picture of the underlying structures. The good ultrasonographer will strive to make his images through an acoustic window.

(Food for thought department: It is not always possible to avoid scanning over bowel; aortic scans, for instance, must be performed through bowel. Although the image is often full of artifacts, it is still useful because we know what the aorta is supposed to look like and therefore we can separate it from the artifacts. The same holds for abdominal masses which are *palpable;* it is possible to scan these masses through bowel because we have some idea of what we are looking for and this enables us to sort out the real echoes from the artifacts. The retroperitoneal lymph nodes are another example of a structure which can be recognized in the presence of artifacts. If there is no clear idea of the type of mass which is being sought, however, we must be very cautious when scanning through bowel. Sometimes an examination is performed to "Rule out abdominal mass": if a "mass" is found on the scan we must be certain that we are not looking at artifacts. Even if the echoes are real, they could always be arising from normal bowel containing feces or fluid. It is permissible to scan through bowel only when an abnormality can be confirmed by some other means, such as physical examination, X-ray, or isotope scan. There are some ultrasonographers who will disagree with us on this point; our opinion is based on a long

series of false diagnoses over several years, however, and we are very concerned with the pitfalls which abound when a scan is produced through bowel. With experience each ultrasonographer will develop his own criteria for when such scans are acceptable.)

OBESITY AND OTHER ANATOMIC PROBLEMS

Before closing this chapter we would like to discuss two items which, while not strictly artifacts, are a major cause of poor images in B-scanning.

The first of these is what we call "bad anatomy." By this we mean anatomic position of the patient's internal organs which makes it difficult or impossible to obtain a good acoustic window. The most common cause of such problems is a small left lobe of the liver. As we shall see, the liver is the main acoustic window in abdominal scanning and a prominent left liver lobe is very helpful for getting a good look at the pancreas. Most patients have good-sized lobes which permit visualizing all but the tail of the pancreas; however, there is a group of people with small left lobes (this is of no clinical significance; livers, like breasts or noses, come in all shapes and sizes). When the left lobe of the liver is small, the stomach occupies the position immediately anterior to the pancreas; and, because there is almost always air in the stomach when the patient is supine, the region of the pancreas often cannot be imaged. Some patients have very narrow livers which permit the transverse colon and its gas to rise up to the level of the pancreas and obscure it. Short, stocky patients are frequently difficult to scan because their livers are located high up under the rib cage and are inaccessible. It is also difficult to scan the kidneys in these patients because the posterior ribs reach nearly to the iliac crest and leave little or no acoustic window.

Most ultrasonographers refer to these situations as "excessive bowel gas" and recommend reexamination after fasting, enemas, or some other maneuver designed to reduce the overall amount of bowel gas. We have also followed this procedure: when an examination is unsatisfactory because there is no acoustic window (or there is "excessive bowel gas"), we sometimes reschedule the patient for another examination. In a few patients a satisfactory scan can be performed at the second sitting; but in the great majority there is no improvement and the pictures look just as they did on the initial examination. The problem is more one of anatomy than excessive gas. If the patient's liver is shaped so that there is no acoustic window, there is little that can be done about it. While we believe that all patients deserve two attempts to have an adequate scan, we also feel that it is not fruitful to persist in scanning such patients in hopes of generating a clinically useful picture.

Fat has a very deleterious effect on the ultrasound beam. The reasons for this are not completely clear, but they probably relate to the multiple interfaces which are present in lipomatous tissue. Fatty tissue is a network of acoustic impedance mismatches which gives rise to numerous, moderately loud echoes. Because of the many interfaces the sound beam is attenuated much more rapidly than is usual, and it is very difficult to get penetration of the beam. Fat also seems to generate significant numbers of internal reverberations, and other factors such as refraction and excessive absorption may also play a part in the loss of beam integrity. For whatever reason, the ultrasonographer quickly learns that fat is his enemy. Skinny patients are very photogenic (or "sonogenic" if you prefer), and the scans obtained from them are beautiful works of art. At the other ex-

treme, very obese patients are impossible to scan; the ultrasound beam is largely attenuated in the subcutaneous fat of the abdominal wall. (On several occasions we have had difficulty in even finding the pregnant uterus in such patients, let alone identifying the placenta or fetal head.) Patients with intermediate amounts of body fat will fall somewhere in between these extremes. There is very little that we can do about the weight of our patients but it is important for us to realize that as the amount of body fat increases, our ability to obtain a good ultrasound picture decreases. The most skilled ultrasonographer in the world cannot generate good pictures in a very obese patient, and even the rank beginner will make beautiful images in a Miss America. The trick is to get the most information possible, given the limits imposed by the body habitus of the patient.

(Mutual interaction department: CT body scanners rely on body fat to produce diagnostically useful images. Because the internal organs all have very similar density when seen by an X-ray beam, it is the presence of internal body fat which helps separate the liver from the pancreas from the bowel. Obese patients produce lovely CT scans while skinny patients yield images which look like a sooty snowball. Thus ultrasound and CT scanning nicely complement each other in their ability to depict the contents of the abdomen.)

Chapter 6

GENERAL SCANNING TECHNIQUES

Did you ever take piano lessons? Dancing lessons? Perhaps you remember physical education classes in school where, for what seemed like an interminable amount of time, you were forced to practice exercises or "fundamentals," as they were called? Our personal experience was with piano lessons. One half of every lesson and one half of every practice session was devoted to technical exercises; scales, arpeggios, finger exercises and the like. The reasoning behind this drudgery eluded us at the time. The teacher said that it was important to learn the technique of piano playing through exercises; they could be practiced over and over until perfected and, while this made the exercise itself unpleasant, it enabled us to acquire the technique to play Chopin with little effort. Now, years later, most of this technique has been forgotten, and today when we try to play Chopin it is tough. Each difficult passage must be struggled over and painstakingly worked out; by the time we are technically able to play the piece we hate it because it was so much work.

B-mode scanning is somewhat the same. A certain amount of technical expertise is required to produce clinically useful scan images; until this technique is mastered scanning is a real hassle. The ultrasonographer must spend so much time and effort in trying to produce a good picture (fiddling with the dials, trying to get the patient in a good position, keeping track of coordinates, remembering to load the camera, dropping the oil can, etc.), that he is unable to concentrate on the real business at hand, which is making a diagnosis or answering a clinical question. Fortunately, the technique of B-mode scanning is not hard to acquire, particularly with gray-scale

scanners and, if the nascent ultrasonographer will spend some time mastering general scanning techniques, he will have no difficulty producing diagnostically useful scans on patients. The material in this chapter represents the scales and arpeggios of B-scanning—the "fundamentals." As such, it is the most important part of the entire text; once the fundamentals are mastered, the ultrasonographer is equipped to perform good examinations and to alter and expand his technique to cope with unusual and difficult scanning techniques.

PATIENT PREPARATION

Nobody enjoys lying in a dirty bed; therefore, before the patient is brought into the examining room, the coverings of the examination table should be changed. If you are using a commercial examination table with a paper cover, this means tearing off the old paper and *neatly* pulling down the new. If you have some other type of table this means changing the sheets and tucking them in *neatly*. In addition to bottom sheets there should be a sheet to cover the lower half of the patient's body and, if the room temperature is less than 72°, a blanket as well. (Remember, the patient does not have much on and is often sick; the ultrasound laboratory is not the place to conserve energy.) Do not forget to change the pillow case and fluff the pillow. Wipe up any old oil, get a clean stack of towels, and tidy up the examining area. Have a step handy so the patient can easily climb onto the table, provide a spot for his personal effects, such as a purse or glasses. (*Little old lady department:* this may sound like a second grade teacher nagging you to keep a clean desk, but it is really important. It takes only a few extra seconds to make the room neat and cheerful and this small investment in time will be amply repaid in good rapport and patient cooperation. An ultrasound examination involves considerable interaction between the patient and ultrasonographer and the more pleasant the procedure is for the patient, the more cooperation the ultrasonographer will receive.)

Before entering the examining room the patient should have changed into a hospital examination gown. How many clothes need be removed depends upon the type of examination. In general, we are aggressive in stripping our patients; we never know when it will be necessary to scan in some unusual plane or through some unforeseen acoustic window. Also the mineral oil we use for a coupling agent seems to find its way onto everything, no matter how carefully we try to contain it, and it is not good to get oil on the patient's clothes. For most abdominal and obstetrical examinations, therefore, we have the patient remove everything but shoes, socks, and bras (pantyhose must go).

Since we begin all but renal examinations in the supine position, the patient is asked to lie on his back on the examination table. A pillow is provided for his head; the lower half of the body is covered with a sheet (and blanket, if necessary), and the examination gown is drawn up to the level of the breasts. Any exposed clothing should be covered with a sheet or disposable drape (such as "Chocks") to protect it from the oil. While doing this, we explain to the patient how the examination will be performed and stress that it is neither dangerous nor uncomfortable.

COORDINATE SYSTEMS

It is important that each laboratory establish a coordinate system for labeling scans. Several different systems have been described and championed by various writers; almost any of them will work as long as everyone who looks at the scans understands it.

It would be nice, however, if some standard could be adopted so that all scans were always oriented the same way, avoiding confusion and making it unnecessary to specify the coordinate system when presenting pictures to other ultrasonographers. The American Institute of Ultrasound in Medicine is in the process of formulating such a standard and will have this task completed by 1978 or 1979. Once this official standard has been adopted, we hope that everyone will use it: in the meantime we offer our own system, which we feel is adequate for most scanning situations and which has the virtue of simplicity.

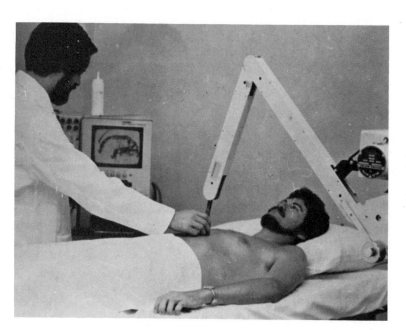

Figure 6–1. The most convenient scanning position for right-handed persons is with the ultrasonographer on the patient's right side and facing him.

First let us consider image orientation. The vast majority of abdominal and pelvic scans are performed with the ultrasonographer on the patient's right, facing the patient's head (Fig. 6–1). This is the most natural position for right-handed persons; it permits easy access to the abdomen and allows the ultrasonographer to face the patient throughout the scan (this is important for good rapport; nobody enjoys looking at someone's back and having an elbow constantly banging his chin). Given this scanning position it is only natural that the scans be oriented with the same perspective; that is, transverse sections should be displayed as if they were viewed from the

A

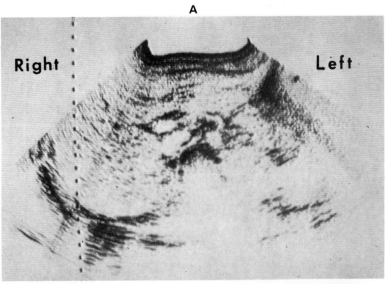

B

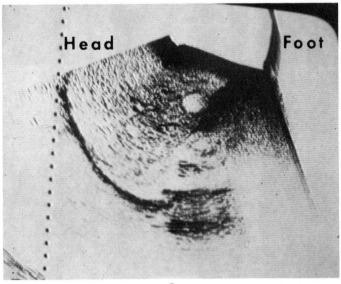

Figure 6–2. The standard orientation of scan images is as if you were looking at the patient from either his right side or from his feet.

A, Proper orientation of a transverse section when the patient is *supine*. The patient's right side is on the viewer's left and the patient's left side is on the viewer's right.

B, Correct orientation for longitudinal sections. The patient's head is on the viewer's left and the patient's feet are on the viewer's right.

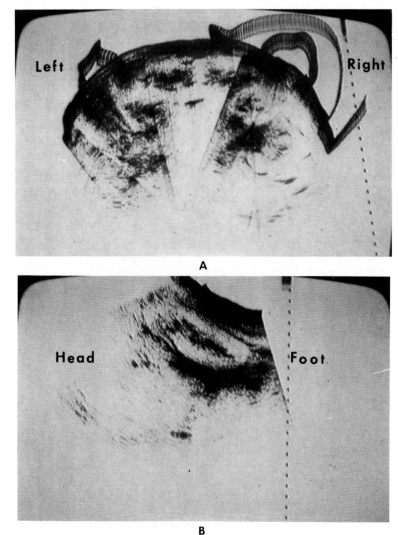

Figure 6–3. When the patient is scanned in the *prone* position, the orientation of the transverse sections will be reversed.

A, Orientation of a transverse scan in the *prone* position. The patient's right is on the viewer's right and the patient's left on the viewer's left.

B, The orientation of the longitudinal section is the same whether the patient is supine or prone — the patient's head is on the viewer's left while the patient's feet are on the viewer's right.

patient's feet and longitudinal scans as if they were viewed from the patient's right side. For transverse sections *in the supine position* this means that the right side of the patient is on the left side of the picture. (Although this is the most common method of displaying images, there are some papers and texts which orient the transverse sections in the opposite manner—as if viewed from the patient's head. Fortunately, this custom is dying out.) For longitudinal sections *in the supine position* the patient's head is displayed on the left side of the picture and his feet on the right side. Figure 6–2 illustrates these displays.

When scanning in the *prone* position there is less agreement as to how the images should be displayed. We prefer to maintain the orientation in which the scan was performed—transverse images as if viewed from the patient's feet and longitudinal pictures with the patient's head to the left side, as shown in Figure 6–3.

Unfortunately, it is not always possible to obtain the desired orientation with gray-scale scanners. Many scanners do not have controls which change the orientation of the display and the only way to switch things around is to move the scanning head to the opposite side of the patient. In a large room, this presents no problems; but, if space is tight, there may be no choice as to scanning head position and picture orientation. (This is no great tragedy since it is quite easy to get used to any orientation with a little experience.)

Next we must consider a coordinate system for labeling the pictures so that we will be able to view them in their proper sequence. Almost everyone agrees that **longitudinal** scans should be related to the midsagittal plane of the body. Therefore we draw a line on the patient right up the middle from the symphysis to the xiphoid. This line represents the "O" longitudinal section; if we make a scan along this line we label it "L,O" meaning "Longitudinal section at the midline." All other longitudinal scans are labeled according to their distance from this line: the right half of the patient is the "positive" side and the left half is the "negative" side. Thus a longitudinal scan 4 centimeters to the right of midline would be labeled "L+4," while a scan 3 centimeters to the left of midline would be marked "L–3." We maintain this convention of the right side of the patient being "positive" and the left side "negative" no matter what position the patient is in; therefore, longitudinal scans of the right side, even in the prone position, would have positive numbers. (We use a slightly different system for renal scans, which we shall discuss in Chapter 8.)

The "O" level for the **transverse** sections is the line connecting the iliac crests. Before beginning the scan we mark this line on the patient's abdomen; a scan along this line would be labeled "C,O" for "Cross-section at the level of the iliac crests." All other transverse scans are identified by their distance from this "O" line; the upper half of the patient is "positive" and the lower half "negative." Thus a scan through the liver, performed 10 centimeters above the iliac crests, would be labeled "C+10," while a scan through the ovaries, performed 6 centimeters below the crests would be marked "C–6." Once again the convention of the upper half of the body being "positive" and the lower half "negative" is maintained, regardless of the position of the patient.

We should point out that not all ultrasonographers use the iliac crests as the "O" level for transverse scans; some use the xiphoid and others the umbilicus. While we have no serious objection to using the xiphoid, we feel that *under no circumstances* should the umbilicus be used as a reference point. The position of the umbilicus is not fixed; it varies from patient to patient and its position is not even constant during the course of the scan unless the patient is lean. Scans performed at different times cannot be compared since changes in the patient's weight will alter its position. As the umbilicus cannot be seen by X-ray, there is no way to correlate its position with X-ray studies or CT pictures. If we seem to be a bit strident on this point, it is because so many publications and lectures present material using the umbilicus as a reference point: this is poor practice and should not be copied. By contrast, the iliac crests are well suited for this role. They are bony landmarks which do not change position, they are readily visible on X-rays and CT scans, and they are located near the center of the abdomen so that both upper abdominal and pelvic scans can be conveniently labeled.

As we mentioned, before we start to scan we draw the two "O" reference lines on the patient's abdomen, as shown in Figure 6–4. During the examination each picture is easily labeled by referring to these lines; this can be done with either a ruler or by using the calibration system included in the scanning head. (*Artist's supply department:* As every ultrasonographer quickly learns, there is no convenient way of marking the patient. All the self-contained markers—"Flair," "Magic-Marker," etc.—are somewhat soluble in oil and may get "washed away" during scanning. Almost any of the solutions used for marking radiotherapy ports are indelible, however, so you may find it convenient to trot down to the radiotherapy department and borrow some of their brew. If there is no radiotherapist at hand, two solutions which work well are Carfusin and Gentian Violet. Both of these come in a bottle and must be applied with a Q-tip. This makes them somewhat inconvenient. Also they are very indelible: this means that if you are sloppy there will be a permanent record on the patient, your hands, your clothes, the machine, or whatever you may have dropped the stuff on. None of the marking solutions can penetrate oil so, if you make marks dur-

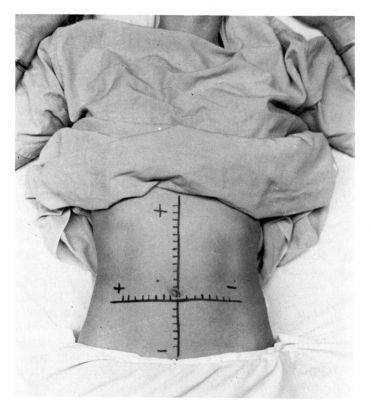

Figure 6-4. The "O" reference lines are the midline (longitudinal sections) and the line through the iliac crests (transverse sections). These lines should actually be drawn on the patient's skin before the examination is started so that when scans are being produced they can be accurately labeled. In this picture we have shown not only the "O" lines, but also some displacements along them. If a scanning plane is displaced toward the patient's head or right side it is considered positive; if the displacement is toward the patient's feet or left side it is negative.

ing a scan—which is frequently a good idea—you must wipe the oil off the patient first.)

The simple coordinate system we have just described has some obvious limitations. First, there is no provision for a scanning plane with is not parallel to one of the "O" lines. Second, there is no way of indicating the angulation of the scanning plane. Finally, the patient's position is not specified. When we began scanning, we had a complicated coordinate system which took all these factors into account, but over the years we have found that keeping track of all these things just was not worth the considerable extra effort involved. In the vast majority of cases the simple "C+3" or "L–7" has proven adequate. Patient position can usually be determined by merely looking at the picture. The skin surface can be seen and, with a knowledge of anatomy, this makes it possible to see whether the patient is prone, supine, upright or decubitus. In those rare cases where confusion would result, it is a simple matter to add a brief notation to the picture such as "sup," "pro," "up," etc.

We have found that only rarely do we use a scanning plane which is not parallel

to one of the "O" lines. This is done in gallbladder scans (as we shall see in Chapter 7, we do not put any coordinates on these scans) and renal scans (for which we have a different system, described in Chapter 8) but almost nowhere else. When it is necessary to describe such a picture, we make a special notation such as "2 cm. below right subcostal line."

We do angle the scanning plane frequently (that is, we scan in planes which are not perpendicular to the top of the examining table). Most of the time this involves longitudinal sections. It is difficult to create a good quality image if the scanning plane is not directed toward the center of the body; therefore, we try to angle the longitudinal sections so that they pass near the spine—the further the section is from the midline, the more the angulation. In these cases it may be useful to specify the angle of the plane as well as the position on the skin where the scan was performed. A vertical scanning plane is considered to have no angulation. When there is an angle involved it is measured as the number of degrees the scan plane differs from the vertical plane (this can be measured on some scanning heads but we usually just "guestimate" it). If the plane is angled toward the "positive" portion of the patient (either the right side or the head) it is considered a positive angle, whereas if the plane is deviated toward the "negative" portion of the patient (the left side or the feet) the angle is considered negative. When we speak of angling the scanning plane toward a specific direction we mean that the sound beam is aimed toward that direction; i.e., if the scanning plane is angled in the positive direction it means that the path of the sound beam is from the feet toward the head or from the left to the right side. Thus, if we perform a longitudinal scan far out on the patient's right side, at 8 centimeters from the midline, for instance, and angle the scan plane so that it passes near the spine, say about a 30° angle, we would label the picture "L+8, −30°." The "L" is for longitudinal, the "+8" means to the right (positive side), and the "−30°" indicates the scanning plane was angled 30° toward the left (negative) side of the patient. Figure 6–5 shows

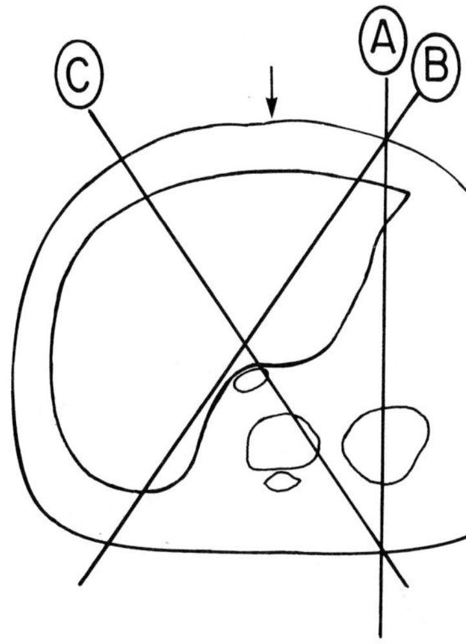

some other examples of the angle notation.

It is important to keep in mind that the number following a "C" or "L" *always* refers to the line where the transducer touches the patient's skin; if there is no angle notation it is assumed that the scanning plane was vertical, that is, perpendicular to the top of the examining table. If the plane is not vertical, then the angle of the plane is added to the notation. (*Quiz time*: We present you with a picture having the following annotation: "C+15, +20°." How was the scanning plane oriented for this scan? Well, let us see. "C" means we are dealing with a cross-section [or transverse section]. The "15" means the transducer was in contact with the patient's skin 15 centimeters from the line through the iliac crests and the "+" means that the 15 centimeters were toward the head [positive direction]. There is an angle number so the scan plane was not vertical; the "20°" indicates the amount of angulation from the vertical while "+" tells us that the angulation was toward the patient's head [positive direction]. Therefore, the scan was performed high in the upper abdomen, 15 centimeters above the iliac crests, and the scan plane was angled 20° toward the head, up under the rib cage. [This scan was probably done to show the pancreas.])

Do not fret if you are having some difficulty coming to grips with this angle notation — you may be able to develop a system of your own which is easier to use. It is important that you not limit yourself to scanning in only the vertical plane, however; there is a considerable amount of diagnostically useful information in other planes as well.

Figure 6–5. A relatively simple angle notation can be used to describe planes which are not vertical. This diagram shows three longitudinal scanning planes and how they would be annotated: the small arrow points to the patient's midline (L,O).

A, "L−4" (When the scanning plane is vertical no angle notation is required.)

B, "L−4, +40°" (The angle with respect to the vertical plane is estimated: if the sound beam passes from the *negative* toward the *positive* side of the patient, the angle is considered positive.)

C, "L+6, −45°" (The sound beam is passing from the *positive* toward the *negative* side of the patient, so the angle is considered negative.)

COUPLING AGENTS

The patient is now on the examining table, fully reassured of the benignity and utility of an ultrasound examination and we have just drawn the two "O" lines on the abdomen, one through the iliac crests and the other up the middle on the line connecting the xiphoid and symphysis. We must now do something about coupling the transducer to the patient. We want to have good acoustic contact between the transducer and the skin so that there will be minimal attenuation of the sound beam.

The most important thing to exclude is air, for, as we saw in Chapter 1, the sound will be totally reflected at an air interface.

The best method of excluding air and providing good sound transmission is to use a liquid between the transducer and the skin. Any liquid will do: water, saline, oil, and aqueous gel are all fine from an acoustic standpoint, but they differ in their convenience. Water and saline dry very quickly and are not viscous so that they are rapidly wiped away by the transducer. This limits their value to the ultrasonographer. Mineral oil does not dry out, is fairly viscous, and resists being wiped away by the transducer. Because it is a good lubricant the transducer can slide smoothly over the skin. Its only disadvantage is the messiness; it is difficult to wipe off and soils clothing. Aqueous gels are easy to clean up and do not damage clothing, but they tend to dry out somewhat and are rather easily wiped away by the transducer. They do not lubricate as well as oil and are much more expensive. Aqueous gels, however, are also more viscous than oil and can provide acoustic coupling over very rough surfaces (when there is lots of body hair, for instance) where oil sometimes fails. We use mineral oil for the bulk of our scanning but keep a small amount of gel on hand for special occasions. The oil is purchased in bulk and dispensed from a plastic squeeze bottle (the kind that is used for ketchup and mustard). If you really want to go first class you can buy a baby bottle warmer to keep the oil at body temperature, but we just warn the patient that the oil will be "a little cold."

The important thing to remember about coupling agents is to use enough. As scanning progresses, the oil or gel is wiped away by the transducer, and acoustic coupling decreases. The change in the picture is subtle; but because of the slowly increasing attenuation, the weaker echoes die out and the picture quality fades away. Failure to use enough coupling agent is one of the most common errors we find in beginning ultrasonographers. From the start, then, we urge you to use lots of oil and reapply it liberally throughout the scan; if the picture quality starts to decrease, the first thing to do is to add more oil. (Now you see why we like to have our patients remove their clothing—if the patient keeps some of his clothes on we tend to skimp on oil, so as not to soil the clothing, and this makes scanning more difficult.)

SCANNING MOTIONS

Now that the patient is well greased, it is time to take the transducer in hand and make a scan. So how shall we move it? There are three basic scanning motions: simple, sector, and compound.

Simple scanning involves moving the transducer in a straight line across the skin without angling the sound beam, as illustrated in Figure 6–6. With the simple scan the sound beam passes over each reflector only once and strikes each interface at only one angle. This is the same scanning motion used by a rectilinear radioisotope scanner or the pick-up head of a tape recorder. (In the latter case it is the tape rather than the head which is moving but the scanning effect is the same.)

Sector scanning involves pivoting the transducer so that the sound beam is rotated about the transducer face, as illustrated in Figure 6–7. The pattern of the sound beam resembles a wedge of pie (known in mathematical circles as a "sector"). This is the type of scanning motion our eyes use as they read a line of print; they start at the left and pivot across the line to the right. Radar also uses a sector scanning motion; we have all seen the radarscope at an airport, rotating in circles as it scans the sky. In sector scanning, as in simple scanning, the sound beam passes over each reflector only once and strikes each interface at only one angle.

Compound scanning is sometimes described as a combination of simple and sector scanning but this is a poor definition. We prefer to consider compound scanning as any scan motion which causes the sound beam to pass over a reflector more than once or causes the beam to strike the interface from more than one angle. Obviously there are many scanning motions which fit this definition. The one most frequently used in B-scanning is the sliding, rocking motion illustrated in Figure 6–8. Compound scanning is the way our eyes evaluate a new car (or an attractive member of the opposite sex) peering up, down, side-to-side and all around. This technique was

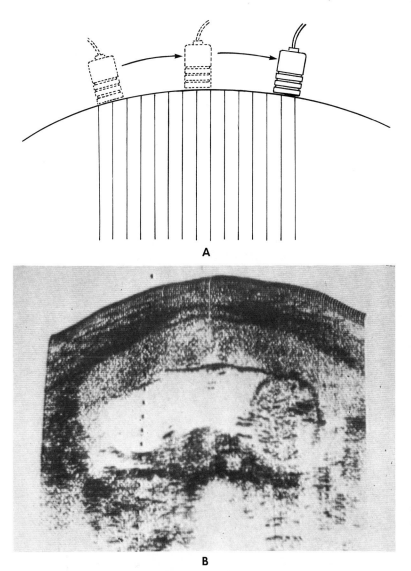

Figure 6-6. In a *simple* scan the transducer is moved in a straight line across the abdomen.
A, Diagrammatic representation of a simple scan. The sound beam passes over each interface only once and strikes each reflector at only one angle.
B, A simple scan of a pregnant uterus.

developed for bi-stable scanning. In Chapter 1 we saw that with bi-stable scanners we are primarily interested in specular echoes—those loud reflections from organ boundaries. Because specular reflections are angle-dependent, it is important that the sound beam strike each interface from several different angles so that the loudest echo will be received. With a bi-stable display it does not matter that the beam passes through some interfaces several times: this distorts the relative amplitudes of the echoes but we are concerned only with the presence or absence of, echoes, not their relative strengths. Gray scale is another matter. When we scan in gray scale we are interested primarily in the small, non-angle-dependent, non-specular echoes; and we want to maintain the correct amplitude relationship between them. For this reason compound scanning is not a suitable technique with gray scale.

THE "SINGLE PASS" SCAN

The correct scanning motion for gray scale is what we call the "single pass" scan;

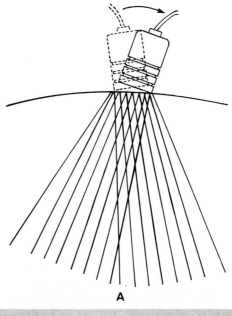

A

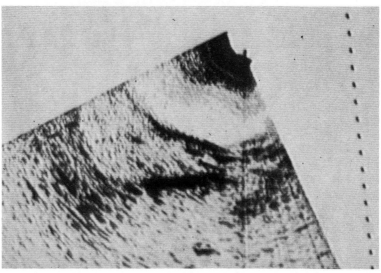

B

Figure 6–7. When the transducer is pivoted about its face a *sector* scan is produced.

A, Diagrammatic representation of a sector scan. The sound beam passes over each interface only once and strikes each reflector at only one angle.

B, A sector scan of a normal female pelvis.

a combination of simple and sector scanning. How the transducer is moved is not especially important as long as two conditions are met: (1) the transducer must always remain over an "acoustic window"; and (2) the sound beam should not pass over any interface more than once.

We discussed the importance of the acoustic window in Chapter 5 and there is no need for further exposition on that point. We want to be certain, however, that everyone understands the importance of

the second point—the sound beam should not pass over an interface more than once. The value of gray-scale scanning rests in its ability to display the relative amplitudes of the echo interfaces; this is what produces the shades of gray and gives the image texture. It is through this texture that the ultrasonographer arrives at a diagnostic decision. (Bi-stable images rely on organ outlines rather than texture for their diagnostic value, as we shall see in Chapter 12.) In order for the texture, or gray scale, to

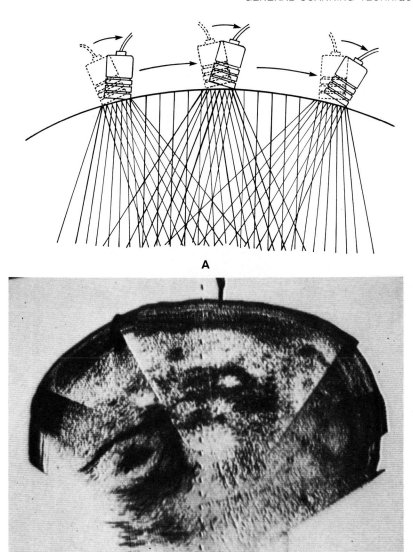

A

B

Figure 6-8. When the transducer is moved so that the sound beam passes over interfaces more than once and strikes reflectors from more than one angle a *compound* scan is produced.

A, Diagrammatic representation of a compound scan.

B, A compound scan of the upper abdomen.

have meaning, each interface must be scanned only one time — each interface gets one chance to produce an echo. If the sound beam passes over interface A once and over interface B two times we can see that, aside from the inherent difference in the two interfaces, B will have a greater chance to produce an echo than A. If interface C is scanned five times it will almost certainly produce a darker echo than if it were scanned only once.

Manufacturers have tried to minimize this effect with circuits to prevent overwriting of the display, as discussed in Chapter 3. These circuits only partially compensate,

however; they can do nothing to affect the echo production and they in no way eliminate the problem. We can demonstrate this easily. Look at Figure 6-9, which is a longitudinal scan through the right lobe of the liver. The scan was begun at the extreme left, the transducer sectored through the liver to the extreme right, then sectored halfway back through the liver: thus, interfaces on the right side of the picture had the sound beam pass over them twice while those on the left were insonated only once. Notice that there are more and darker echoes on the right side of the picture than on the left. This is a normal liver, and there

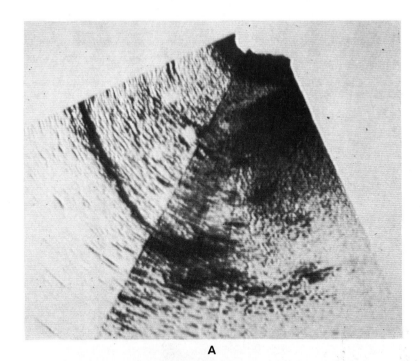

A

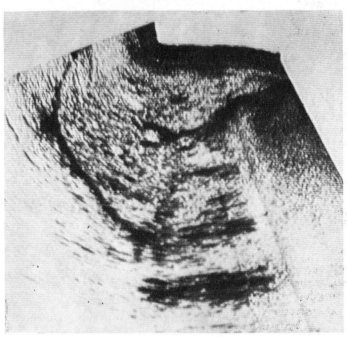

B

Figure 6–9. Passing the sound beam over an interface more than once distorts the gray scale.
A, A longitudinal scan through the right lobe of the liver. The sound beam was started on the left and swept across the liver to the right and then swept half way back: the interfaces on the right half of the picture are darker than those on the left and there is an artifactual boundary in the liver.
B, The same scan as in A, except that the sound beam was passed over the liver only once. The echoes have the same intensity and it is easy to see that the liver is normal.

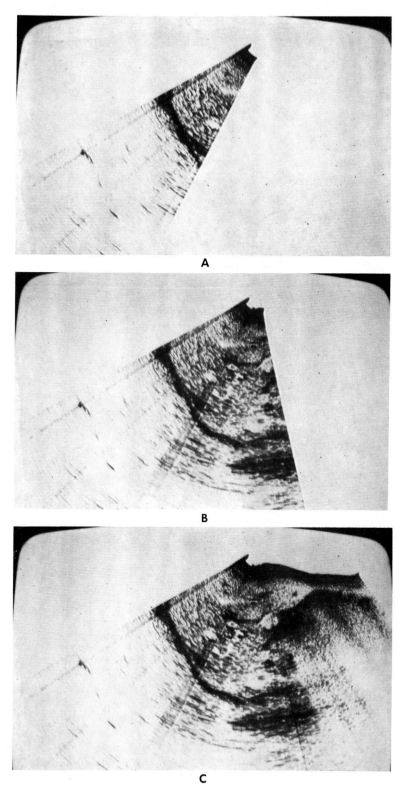

Figure 6-10. Gray scale requires a *single pass* scan technique. The buildup of a single pass scan is shown in pictures *A*, *B*, and *C*; this is a longitudinal scan through the right lobe of the liver.

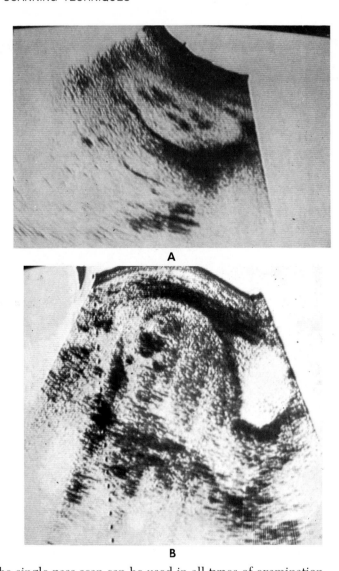

A

B

Figure 6–11. The single pass scan can be used in all types of examination.
A, Longitudinal scan of a normal kidney.
B, A uterus with a leiomyoma (notice the calcifications and shadowing).

Legend continued on opposite page.

is no real difference between the interfaces on the right side and those on the left, yet note how different the picture is. This difference represents an artifact introduced by the scan technique. Good scanning technique requires "equality of opportunity"—that is, every interface should have the same opportunity to produce an echo as its neighbor: this is possible only if the sound beam is passed over each interface once and once alone.

There are many ways to produce a single pass scan—usually it involves a sort of sliding, sector motion. The transducer is aimed at one side of the image and sectored until it is aimed approximately at the center of the patient; it is then moved over the skin surface until the end of the acoustic window is reached. The transducer is not moved off the window; instead it is again sectored. Figure 6–10 shows the progression of a single pass scan. This process is somewhat difficult to describe and the best way to get a feel for it is to practice some scans—you will quickly get the knack. The entire scan motion should consist of a single smooth sweep. The hardest part is staying over the acoustic window, but, if you watch the image as it is built up on the TV screen, you will be able to tell when the

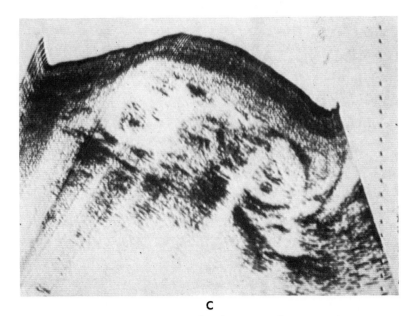

C

Figure 6–11 Continued. C, A normal pregnancy.

transducer reaches the edge of the window. (There is no harm in moving off the window as long as you realize the limited value of the resulting image.)

The single pass technique is quite easy to master when performing obstetrical, pelvic, renal, and longitudinal abdominal scans, as the only difficulty in these situations is finding an acoustic window. When the acoustic window is large (as occurs over the right lobe of the liver or the pregnant uterus), the scan may have a good deal of sliding with only limited sectoring required. When the acoustic window is small (as occurs when scanning over the left lobe of the liver, between ribs, or in a pelvic scan when the bladder is only partially filled), the entire scan may have to be sectored. Figure 6–11 shows different types of single pass scans.

TRANSVERSE ABDOMINAL SCANS

Transverse scans of the upper abdomen are the most difficult to perform with a single pass technique, in fact, the majority of transverse pictures which are published were made with a compound rather than a single pass motion. There is a natural instinct to scan the entire abdominal wall (somehow the picture seems incomplete unless the transducer is moved completely across the body from one flank to the

other). This is a powerful urge — we have to fight it every time we make a scan; but it is important that it be suppressed. Moving the transducer across the abdomen from flank to flank does produce a lovely picture of the skin and abdominal wall — unfortunately these structures are not important diagnostically. We are concerned with internal organs and masses and the image of these structures is degraded by the flank-to-flank scan. There are two reasons for this: (1) It is impossible to stay over an acoustic window using this technique; the beam, of necessity, will pass through some ribs and bowel. (2) Since the beam is directed toward the center of the patient, it is inevitable that some interfaces near the center of the body will be scanned more than once.

Good transverse scans of the abdomen are made with the single pass technique. The acoustic window may vary, depending on what particular area of the abdomen is under investigation. For most purposes we make a single pass between the costal margins. We start with the transducer against the patient's right costal edge and angled steeply to the patient's right; the transducer is then swung back toward the center of the patient and over toward the left side until the left costal margin is encountered; the scan is completed by sectoring the transducer to the extreme left side of the patient (assuming of course that we are still located over an acoustic window).

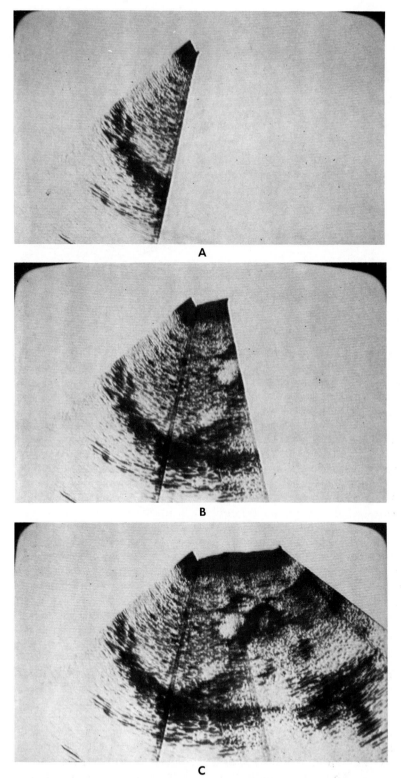

A

B

C

Figure 6–12. Single pass scanning is just as important with transverse sections as it is with longitudinal ones. Pictures *A*, *B*, and *C* show the sequential buildup of a single pass transverse scan of the upper abdomen.

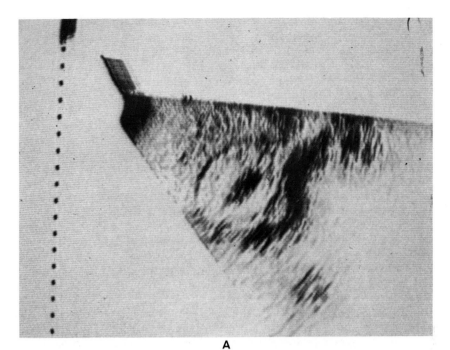

A

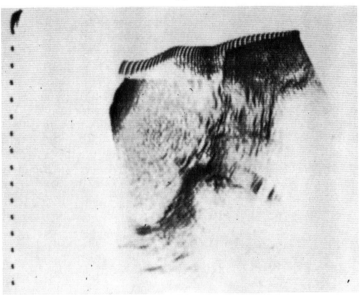

B

Figure 6–13. When the acoustic window is small a single pass scan may consist of only a sector motion.

 A, The right kidney and retroperitoneum in cross section. The patient was supine and the transducer was placed between two ribs and sectored.

 B, The normal spleen as seen by a sector scan between two ribs. The patient was lying on his right side.

Figure 6–12 illustrates this process. Naturally the higher the scan is performed the more sectoring will be required: up near the xiphoid the entire scan may consist of a single sector motion.

 Scanning between the costal margins will give the best image of the central abdominal structures; the great vessels, pancreas, central liver, biliary tree, gallbladder, and para-aortic nodes. In skinny patients it will also produce good pictures of the right retroperitoneum and occasionally the left retroperitoneum (if there is something to displace the overlying bowel). It usually will not give a good picture of the spleen (see Chapter 7 for hints on scanning the spleen) and, in large patients, the retroperitoneal areas will not be well visualized because the interfaces are so far from the transducer that their echoes are lost by attenuation. To see these deep areas we must get the transducer closer to them. How do we go about that? We simply pick a different acoustic window—one that is closer to the area of interest. If we are interested in the right kidney and retroperitoneum we will select a point on the right flank (in between the ribs, of course) and make a sector scan from there. If the spleen is what we seek, we will roll the patient up on his right side and make a sector scan between two left posterior ribs (Fig. 6–13). A knowledge of anatomy is all that is required to select the best transducer position for imaging a specific area.

If it is necessary to use more than one acoustic window to make a complete image, each transducer pass may be placed on the same picture as long as they do not overlap significantly. (If there were significant overlap we would only need to make a single pass anyway.) Figure 6–14 shows how a complete transverse image of the abdomen can be made using only the single pass scanning technique. Of course, you have noticed that the single pass pictures do not give a complete view of the body wall. While at first glance this makes the picture less appealing (because we all like to have a complete image of the cross-section of the body on every transverse scan),

it does not affect its diagnostic utility. The single pass technique makes good images of what is important—the internal anatomy.

RESPIRATION

Any movement of the interfaces during the scan degrades the resolution and image quality. There are four causes of motion: (1) patient respiration; (2) motion from the beating heart and pulsing blood vessels; (3) motion due to the pressure of the transducer; and (4) involuntary motion of the patient (such as a tremor or seizure). There is nothing we can do about causes (2) and (4); fortunately involuntary patient motion is rare and cardiac-induced movements are small (except for the heart and aorta, of course). Motion caused by transducer pressure is uncommon in abdominal scanning unless the patient is quite flabby and the ultrasonographer is really digging in with the transducer. The scan should be performed with only enough pressure to maintain good skin contact. (*Off-limits department:* When scanning very malleable organs, such as the breasts, the motion introduced by transducer pressure is significant. For this reason it is not possible to make good contact scans of these organs.)

Respiratory motion causes significant displacement of the upper abdominal organs—as much as 4 to 5 centimeters. Therefore, we ask the patient to hold his breath while the scan is being performed.

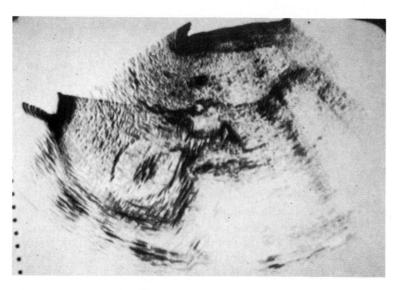

Figure 6–14. If the entire abdomen cannot be seen on one transducer sweep it is permissible to move the transducer and make another single pass scan on the same picture *providing* that the two images do not overlap. In this example the anterior portion of the abdomen was seen with a scan between the costal margins, and the right kidney and retroperitoneum were filled in with another single pass scan between the ribs. The left half of the abdomen contained only artifacts.

Since a single pass scan takes only 2 or 3 seconds this is no problem except for extremely ill patients. We almost always have the patient hold his breath in deep inspiration; this has three advantages: (1) Since there is more air in the lungs, most people feel more comfortable in inspiration than expiration. (2) Many patients perform a Valsalva maneuver in deep inspiration; this distends the venous structures of the abdomen and makes them easier to identify. (3) The liver, gallbladder, and kidneys are displaced downward into the abdomen during inspiration. This provides a much larger acoustic window and greatly facilitates scanning the upper abdomen and kidneys. Flexibility must be maintained; however, occasionally the area of interest will be better seen on a scan in expiration or partial inspiration.

Respiratory motion has little effect on the pelvic organs so it is not necessary to have the patient hold her breath during obstetrical or pelvic scans.

SCANNING PLANES

Although the vertical scanning plane (that is, the plane perpendicular to the table top) is most frequently used, it is by no means always the best. The great majority of transverse scans are done vertically; but when making longitudinal images, it is useful to keep the scanning plane oriented roughly through the center of the patient,

as shown in Figure 6–15. This has two benefits. First, it is easier to maintain good acoustic contact between the transducer face and skin; and second, the sound beam is more nearly perpendicular to the large specular interfaces.

Sometimes it is necessary to angle the scanning plane to make use of acoustic windows. For example, the symphysis pubis is above the cervix and hence, if a transverse scan through the cervix is desired, it is necessary to angle the scan plane toward the feet (in the negative direction)—the transducer will remain above the symphysis and the beam will be angled underneath the bone to the cervix. In short patients, the pancreas may be located high up under the rib cage where it can be visualized on transverse section only when the scanning plane is angled toward the head (positive direction). In Chapter 8 we shall discuss angling the scanning plane to visualize the kidneys. The aorta and adrenals are sometimes best seen when the scan is performed in the frontal plane, that is, a plane perpendicular to the midsagittal and vertical transverse planes; we shall discuss this further in Chapter 7.

SCAN INTERVALS

We cannot give any hard and fast recommendations as to how far apart scans should be spaced; this depends to a large extent on the individual examination. If the purpose of the examination is to rule out gallstones and on the first scan a gallstone is seen, then the study may be over. On the other hand, gallstones cannot be excluded unless the gallbladder has been examined at 5 mm. intervals! If the request is "Evaluate nature of palpable abdominal mass," only a few scans may be required to say that the mass is cystic or non-cystic. Then again the mass may be found to be much larger than what is palpated, and many sections may be required to completely define it. The point to keep in mind is flexibility. There is no "standard" scanning routine. Each examination must be structured to answer the clinical question which has been raised. For this reason, instead of giving scanning formulas, we shall explore various methods of answering specific questions. *The correct number of scans for an exami-*

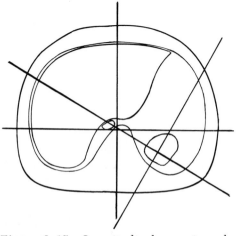

Figure 6–15. Longitudinal scanning planes should be angled so that they pass near the center of the body.

nation is that number which allows the ultrasonographer to arrive at a diagnostically useful decision. We feel very strongly that the physician who will interpret the examination must see the pictures and be satisfied that the clinical questions have been answered *before* the patient leaves the ultrasound laboratory.

SCANNER CONTROLS

Proper scanning technique is vital for producing good images, but the best of techniques will be worthless if the scanner is not properly adjusted. Although the scanning console may appear quite foreboding at first glance, there are actually only a few adjustments to be made. (This represents a major improvement over early bi-stable instruments, the control panel of which resembled that of a 747 jet.) If you skipped Chapter 3, where we examined how the major controls work, we suggest you go back and read it before continuing; otherwise you may find this discussion a little hard to follow.

Let us quickly dispense with three controls which should be set once and forgotten: the **near gain suppression**, the **reject**, and the **enhance.** Depending on the manufacturer and model, your scanner may or may not have the first two of these. If they are present, turn them both off. Neither near gain suppression nor reject is used in B-mode abdominal and pelvic scanning. As we saw in Chapter 3, these controls eliminate real echoes as well as artifacts. Although they may make the image appear "prettier," their use cuts down on the quantity of the data available and diminishes the diagnostic utility of the scan. We prefer to have all the signals, both echoes and artifacts, preserved on the image and use our own judgment to decide what is real and what is not. All gray-scale scanners have an enhance knob. It is not particularly important where this is set as long as it is not changed. Most ultrasonographers, including us, leave the enhance in the middle of its range; this is a matter of personal taste, however; and you should probably experiment some before making your own decision. Once you have picked a setting, stick with it. There are enough variables in B-mode scanning already; we do not need to add any others.

Next we should adjust the **centering.** All scanners have a button which, when pressed, centers the TV display at the position of the transducer. After the patient is in place and the scanning head has been positioned in the correct plane, the transducer should be placed over the center of the area to be scanned. With the transducer in this position the centering button is pressed; the position monitor is now aligned so that the image will be displayed in the center of the TV screen. (The "zoom" control must be switched off, otherwise the centering will be controlled by the position of the joystick.) We will have to repeat this procedure every time the scanning head or the patient is moved. (*Absent-minded department:* We all forget to do this occasionally: if you are trying to make a scan and nothing appears on the TV, try pressing the "center" button—this will usually rectify the situation.)

There are two ancillary controls associated with the centering which adjust the position of the centering dot on the TV display. These are usually labeled "horizontal" and "vertical" corresponding to their effect on the position of the dot. For the great majority of scans we want this dot located in the middle of the TV screen and about 1 centimeter below the top edge. (It is a simple matter to adjust this: we simply move the "horizontal" and "vertical" controls until the dot is in the desired position.) When we scan the gallbladder in the upright position we will move the dot so that it is midway between the top and bottom of the TV screen and is 1 centimeter from the right edge. This is another of those concepts which are difficult to describe but will be quite easy to grasp when you start working with the machine.

The next step is to select a **scale** for the scans. All scanners have a set of pushbuttons on the console corresponding to various scales: 1:1, 2:1, and 3:1 are universal and some machines also offer 4:1 and 1/2:1. Most abdominal scans can be done on 3:1, but very large patients and late term pregnancies may require a 4:1 scale if the whole patient is to be included on a single picture. We use the 2:1 and 1:1 scales when we want a larger image of an area in question (as we saw in Chapter 3, this is preferable to enlarging a picture with the "zoom"). Due to physical limitations of scan converters, it is technically difficult to scan on the 1:1 scale so we usually confine our magnification to 2:1. We must always remember to flash in the scale markers on each image so that there will be a permanent record on the pictures.

The **zoom** control has little utility and we leave it turned off most of the time. Although we occasionally use the joystick to correct poor centering of the image, we never use the magnification (except to impress hospital trustees with the versatility of the machine).

The **TV monitor used for viewing** the image has four standard television controls: contrast, brightness, vertical hold, and horizontal hold. These can be adjusted as necessary to give a pleasing image to the eye. We like to turn the contrast up until "snow" appears in the picture and then back it off slightly. The brightness level will depend on the amount of background light in the examining room; the greater the light, the higher the brightness must be set. The TV monitor used for hard copy also has these controls—we shall discuss how they should be set in a moment.

Gain and TCG

Gain and TCG are the two most important controls on the scanner, as they require continuous adjustment during the course of the scan. Let us consider the TCG first.

The purpose of **TCG** is to give a balanced picture; it is correctly adjusted when the density of echoes is the same throughout the image. If the echoes in the near field are, in general, darker than those in the far field, the TCG is too low. If the far field echoes are darker than the near field ones, the TCG is too high. Every TCG control has some kind of scale associated with it, and in the past some manufacturers have given "recommendations" as to where the TCG should be set for different types of examinations. These recommendations are about as useful as a hole in the head. There is no way to predict what amount of TCG will be needed since this depends on the characteristics of the transducer and the type of tissue through which the beam is traveling. The only correct way to adjust this control is by eye. If the far field echoes are weak, turn up the TCG; if the near field

is washed out, turn it down. As shown in Figure 6–16, the goal is uniform echo density throughout the picture. (*Know your machine department:* Some scanners have a single TCG control while others have a series of controls. The same principles apply to either. The multiple controls give greater flexibility in balancing the echo density but are less convenient to use.)

Once the TCG is adjusted the **gain** must be set. For convenience we shall assume that all machines have a single gain control (the attenuator). This may be labeled "gain" or "output" or "sensitivity"—consult the instruction manual of your scanner to find out which. If there is more than one gain control (as was common in older scanners) adjustments should be made in only one. (We prefer to use the attenuator to adjust the gain.) Consult the instruction manual to find the location of the gain and TCG controls on your particular scanner.

The gain determines the overall echo density of the picture—it is analogous to the volume control on a stereo system; when the gain is increased all of the echoes become darker; when it is decreased they all become lighter. With gray-scale scanning we want to display *every* echo; we will separate them on the basis of their relative amplitudes. Therefore, the gain should be adjusted so that echoes are received from *all* organs and tissues. The only white areas on the scan should be fluid-filled structures such as the gallbladder, bladder, aorta, amniotic cavity, or cysts. Solid tissues should never be echofree—if they are, the gain is set too low. This is by far the most common error in setting the scanner controls. Almost all beginning ultrasonographers scan at too low a gain, producing a light gray liver and white kidneys. Echoes which are not displayed are worthless for diagnostic purposes. The main advantage of a gray-scale scanner is its ability to record *all* echoes on a single scan; if the gain is so low that some echoes are not recorded, much of the value of the gray-scale scan is lost. When the gain is properly set, the liver and placenta should be medium to dark gray, the kidneys and spleen should be light gray and the normal pancreas should be nearly black. Of course, the capsule of the liver and kidneys and the walls of major vessels will be totally

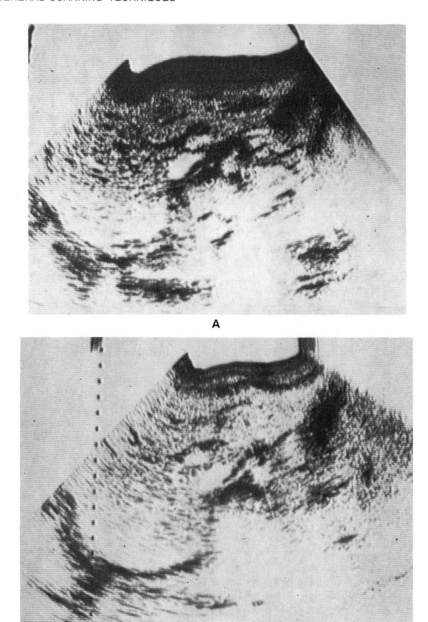

A

B

Figure 6–16. The TCG controls must be set so that the echoes from the near field and far field are in balance.

A, The TCG is too low. The near field echoes are too dark while those in the far field are too light. If the gain is increased to fill in the distant areas the anterior portion of the scan will be obscured with artifacts.

B, The same scan as in *A* except that the TCG is now properly adjusted: there is good balance between the echoes of the near and far fields.

Legend continued on the opposite page.

black since these are large, specular echoes, many times the magnitude of the parenchymal echoes.

Unfortunately, as the gain is increased, artifacts increase, and thus there is a point of diminishing return; that is, at some point a further increase in gain results in the generation of more artifacts than real echoes. The ultrasonographer's job is to find that point and set the gain control so that he

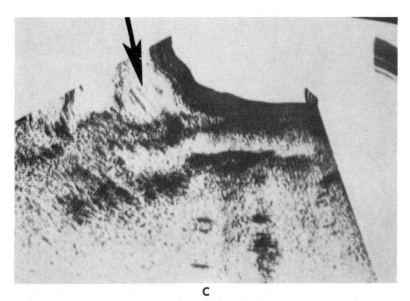

C

Figure 6–16 Continued. C, A longitudinal scan through the aorta with the TCG too high: there are not enough echoes in the liver (*arrow*), yet the underlying aorta is beginning to fill with artifacts.

displays the maximum number of real echoes with a minimum of artifacts. This takes skill. Because it is easier to recognize when the gain is set too low than when it is too high, we suggest that the scan be started at a relatively low level and the gain increased until the proper point is found. Figures 6–17 through 6–19 show examples of correct and incorrect gain settings.

TRANSDUCER SELECTION

In general we want to use a transducer of as high a frequency as possible to give maximum resolution. However, owing to the considerable attenuation in the abdomen and the limited capacity of the TCG amplifier, it is often desirable to use lower-frequency transducers with abdominal

scans. Figure 6–20 illustrates such a case. The TCG is turned all the way up, yet the echoes from deep in the liver are still weak. If the gain is increased to compensate for this, the near field is filled with artifacts. There are two ways to handle this situation. First, we could make two separate pictures; one at moderate gain for the near field and the second at very high gain for the far field. The other method is to switch to a lower frequency transducer, 1.6 MHz, for example. The lower frequency undergoes less attenuation and there is better beam penetration so the TCG amplifier is able to compensate. The overall gain can therefore be reduced, and this decreases the number of artifacts. Thus, for a small sacrifice in resolution, we have gained a significant improvement in overall image quality and a considerable reduction in artifacts.

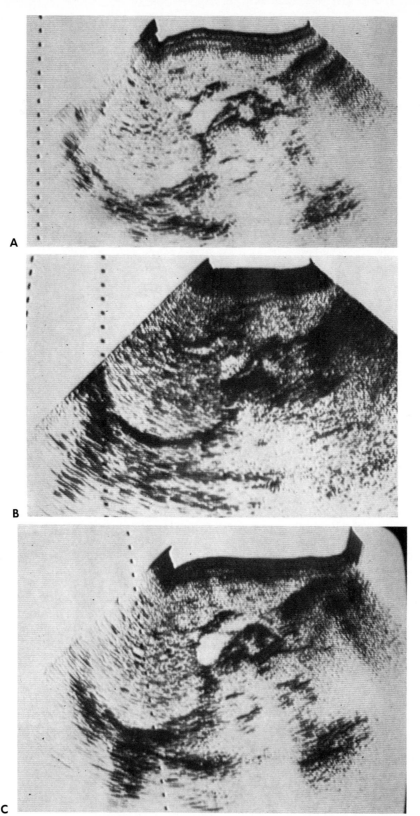

Figure 6–17. The gain control must be set so that echoes are received from all solid tissue — echoes which are not recorded have no diagnostic value.

A, The gain is too low; there are too few echoes in the liver to make any diagnostic decision.

B, The same picture as in *A* but with the gain set too high; too many artifacts are produced with too high a gain.

C, The same picture as in *A* but with the gain set just right; there is good echo density in the liver but not too many artifacts.

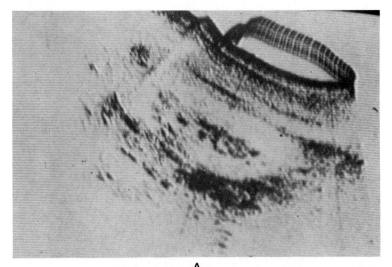

A

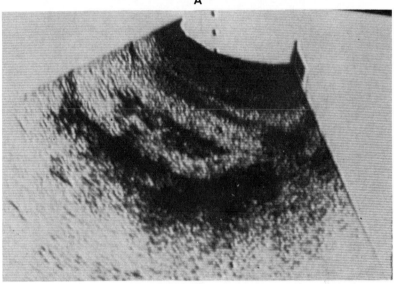

B

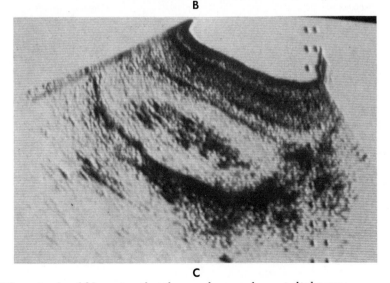

C

Figure 6-18. The gain should be set so that the renal parenchyma is light gray.
A, Longitudinal section of kidney with gain too low; a small renal cyst would be missed.
B, The same picture as in *A* except gain is now too high; there are too many artifacts.
C, The same picture as in *A* except with the gain correctly set.

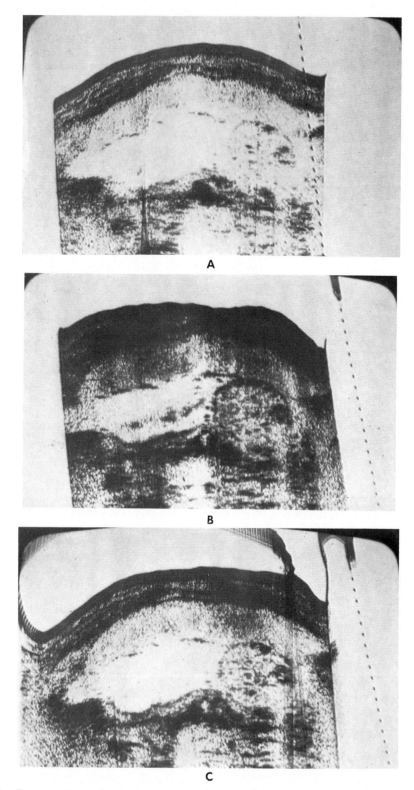

Figure 6–19. Proper gain setting is important in obstetrical scans.
A, The gain is too low; placental texture and fetal anatomy cannot be seen.
B, The same picture as in A except gain is set too high; there are too many artifacts.
C, The same picture as in A except the gain is set just right.

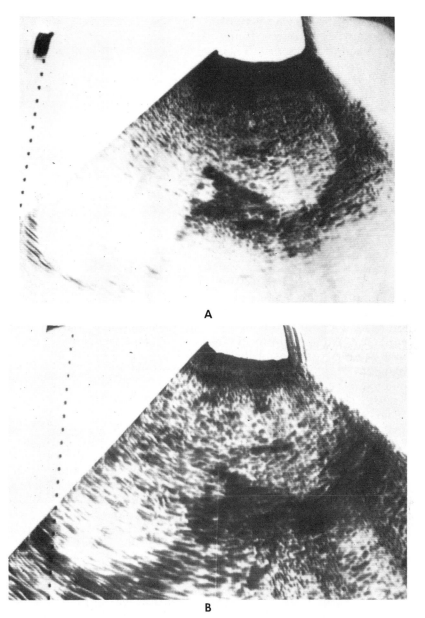

A

B

Figure 6–20. Lower frequency transducers, while having slightly poorer resolution than higher frequency models, often produce better images because of their superior penetration.

A, A transverse scan of the abdomen made with a 2.25 MHz transducer. The TCG is set to maximum but, due to high attenuation in the liver, no echo information is available in the far field.

B, The same picture as in *A* except that a 1.6 MHz transducer has been used. The lower frequency is attenuated less and the penetration of the sound beam is improved.

In some situations, where information about interfaces 10 or more centimeters deep is desired, it is impossible to scan with any but a low-frequency transducer. Frequencies greater than 2.5 MHz are totally attenuated at this depth, and no matter how high the gain no echoes will be re-ceived. On the other hand, when scanning superficial structures, attenuation is not a problem and higher-frequency transducers (3.5 MHz or 5.0 MHz) can be used.

It takes some experience to know which transducers will give the best picture in a specific situation. We usually start all our abdominal and obstetrical examinations with a 2.25 MHz transducer. If there is any difficulty seeing deep structures or if we are plagued with artifacts because very high gain is needed, we switch to a 1.6 MHz transducer. If an area of interest is 4 to 8 centimeters from the skin, we may switch to a 3.5 MHz transducer for a more precise look.

HARD COPY

There is nothing more frustrating than working your tail off to get a good scan and then having the pictures come out looking as if they had been developed in 4-day-old dishwater. Coupling the hard-copy system to the TV monitor is a tricky business and takes considerable effort if the pictures are to look as good as the image on the screen. Little attention has been paid to this in the past: most ultrasonographers shrug their shoulders, curse the inadequacies of Polaroid film, and dream of getting one of the expensive "automatic" cameras. As an old Roman once said: "The fault, dear Brutus, is not in our stars, but in ourselves." If we will take the time to calibrate the camera with the TV monitor we can make good pictures even with the simple old Polaroid camera.

(Sit down and relax — we need to indulge in a few moments of basic physics of film: we promise to keep it brief.) The behavior of film emulsion when it is struck by light can be described by what is known as an "I & D" curve. A simplified form of this curve is illustrated in Figure 6–21. The horizontal axis shows the **intensity** (or brightness) of the light striking the film; we have calibrated it in arbitrary units, 1 through 10. Now this light causes the emulsion to turn black. The **density** (or "blackness") of the emulsion is plotted on the vertical axis in arbitrary units I through X. The I & D curve (what does I & D stand for?) shows how dark the emulsion will become after exposure by a certain amount of light. In the example in Figure 6–21, 3 units of light would give a density of II, while 7 units of light would yield a density of VIII. Naturally the more light the greater the density. Notice that the curve is nearly a straight line over much of its length, but that it levels out at each end. (*Black is white department:* The emulsion of most films,

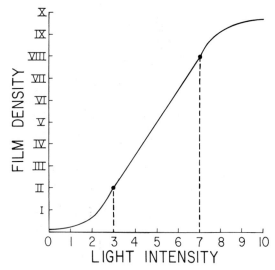

Figure 6–21. An I & D curve shows the relationship between the amount of light striking the film and the density ("blackness") produced by the emulsion. As the light intensity increases, so does the film density. For the film illustrated here, 3 units of light will give a density of II while 7 units of light will yield a density of VIII.

including 70 mm and X-ray film, turns black when struck by light. Polaroid film behaves in just the opposite manner — it starts out black and turns white when struck by light. In the following discussion you should think of "density" as "blackness" if you are using X-ray or 70 mm film and as "whiteness" if using Polaroid film.)

Each film has a characteristic I & D curve which describes its behavior. Look at Figure 6–22 where the curves of two different films, W and X, are compared. The slopes of the lines are the same, but their position is different. It takes more light to produce the same density in film X than in film W. Another way to look at this is to say that the same exposure — 4 units of light, for example — will make film W darker than film X. (*Advanced Placement Test:* Part I. *Question:* What does this say about the relative "speeds" or ASA numbers of the two films? *Answer.* Since it takes less light to expose W, W is "faster" or has a higher ASA number than X.) If we were using film W to make our hard copy, we would have to expose it less — by turning down the monitor brightness, or changing the f-stop of the camera — than if we were using film X.

Now look at Figure 6–23 where we compare two more films, Y and Z. The difference in these films is the slope of the line. A small change in light exposure – 2 units, for example – will cause a greater change in density in film Z than in film Y. (*Advanced Placement Test:* Part II. *Question:* Which film has more "contrast"? *Answer:* Since the density of Z changes more quickly than Y, Z has more contrast. Small changes in exposure will make large changes in the density.)

You are probably wondering what all this has to do with making good hard copy. Well, simply this: in order to make an accurate photograph of what is on the TV screen, the contrast and brightness of the monitor must be set so that they match the I & D curve of the film being used. Consider Figure 6–23 once again. Let us suppose that the contrast and brightness controls on the TV monitor are set so that the very darkest area on the screen has a brightness of 2 units and the very lightest area a brightness of 9 units. If we were using film Y we would have a good match; the I & D curve would nicely cover our brightness range. But suppose we were using film Z. The match is now poor.

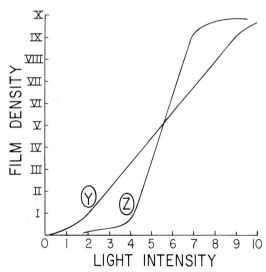

Figure 6–23. The two films shown here have different slopes and hence are of different "contrast." Film Y changes density more slowly than film Z and is a lower contrast film than Z.

Echoes at either end of the scale, say, for example, those which produced 2, 3 and 4 or 7, 8 and 9 units of light on the TV, would look the same on the film. The picture would be too contrasty, and we would have lost the very weakest and very loudest echoes.

The other extreme is also undesirable. Suppose that we now set the TV monitor so that the range of brightness is 4 to 7 units of light. This gives a good match with film Z, but what if we were using film Y? We would not lose any echoes but we might have a hard time separating them since they would all be displayed in medium gray densities IV to VI. Our picture would look as if it had been taken through the Great London Fog of 1893.

So where do we set things? Under ideal circumstances we would try to match the film I & D curve exactly. Unfortunately, circumstances are not ideal (are they ever?). The TV monitor used for hard copy drifts; that is, it changes its brightness spontaneously. The film I & D curve also varies slightly between batches of film (this is a greater problem with Polaroid film than with X-ray or 70 mm film). The curve is also affected by the conditions under which

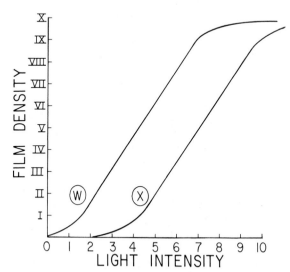

Figure 6–22. The slope of the I & D curve determines the "contrast" of a film while its position determines the "speed." The two films illustrated here have the same slope and hence the same contrast. Film W is "faster" than film X, however: 4 units of light give a density of V on film W, but a density of only I on film X.

the film is developed. Finally, every time an image is copied the contrast will increase. Because we must allow leeway for all these factors, we shall try to set the TV monitor to the middle portion of the I & D curve, encompassing about two-thirds of the slope as shown by the dashed lines in Figure 6–21.

TV MONITOR CONTROLS

There are at least two TV monitors on gray-scale scanners. We discussed the controls for the viewing monitor earlier and now we will consider the hard-copy monitor. Our goal is to hit the middle portion of the I & D curve of the film, but how do we find where that is? We will use the scientific process known as trial and error.

We start by putting the gray-scale test pattern on the screen (consult the instruction manual of your machine to do this). We take a picture and look at the results. We want to have the darkest gray level (corresponding to the loudest echoes) appear nearly, but not quite, black while the lightest gray level (corresponding to the softest echoes) is almost, but not quite, white. We must play around with the "contrast" and "brightness" controls on the monitor until the picture comes out like that.

It takes a good deal of time, patience, and film to arrive at the proper settings. Set aside two or three hours when you start. Things go fastest if you move only one control at a time: start with the "contrast"; and when you are satisfied with the spread of the gray bars, adjust the overall appearance with the "brightness." For some reason the contrast and brightness controls are closely linked and changing one usually produces a small change in the other as well. It will, therefore, take some juggling to get them both properly set.

The overall brightness of the picture can also be controlled by changing the f-stop or shutter speed of the camera. The f-stop controls the amount of light reaching the camera lens. When the f-stop number is increased, *less* light reaches the film and the overall picture density decreases. If the f-stop number is made smaller, *more* light reaches the film and picture density increases. Changing the f-stop does not affect the contrast of the image, and, therefore, we like to make the final brightness adjustments this way rather than with the brightness control. The amount of light reaching the film can also be controlled by varying the shutter speed—the shorter the shutter speed, the less light and the less dense the final image. The shutter speed should not be *shorter* than 1/4 second, however; shorter speeds than this will not allow the TV beam to complete its scan and will produce a dark line (known as a scan bar) in the picture. Figures 6–24 and 6–25 show examples of correct and incorrect monitor settings.

Now that we have the monitor controls set, we surely do not want anyone to change them. Signs, warnings, electric fences, and guard dogs will work temporarily, but eventually somebody will ignore these and change the settings—"just trying to improve the picture"—and there will go two hours of work down the drain. The best way to protect the controls is to take the knobs off once you have set them: in many machines they just pull straight out, in others you must loosen a set screw. (*Gadgeteering department:* An even better solution to this problem is replacing the stock controls with calibrated potentiometers which can be locked. Your in-house electronics repairman should be able to do this for you. These calibrated "pots" have two advantages: (1) They can be locked in position, and (2) the calibration allows you to easily retrieve a setting if someone changes it. If you are using more than one type of hard copy—Polaroid and X-ray film for example—each will require different settings, and the ability to return to precise settings of brightness and contrast is vital.)

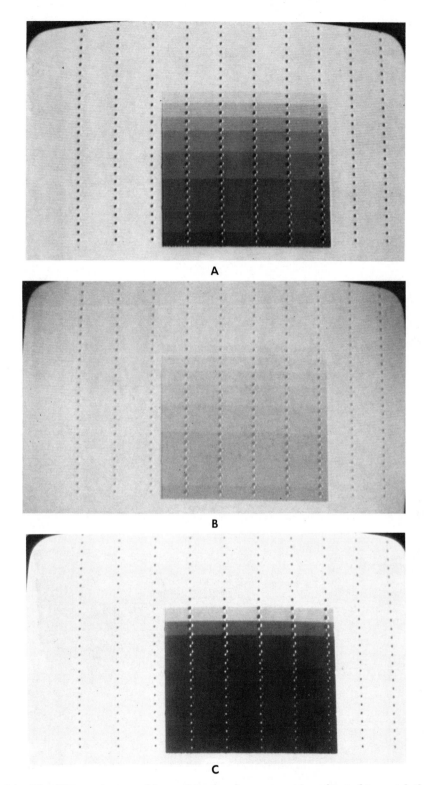

Figure 6-24. The TV monitor used for making hard copy must be adjusted to match the film being used.

A, A photograph of the gray scale standardization bars with the contrast set too high: most of the gray shades are lost and the image is essentially composed of two tones—white and black.

B, The same picture as in *A* but with the contrast set too low: although all eight shades of gray are recorded it is very difficult to distinguish between them.

C, The same picture as in *A* but with the contrast set correctly: all eight shades of gray are recorded; the darkest shade is almost, but not quite, black, while the lightest shade is almost, but not quite, white.

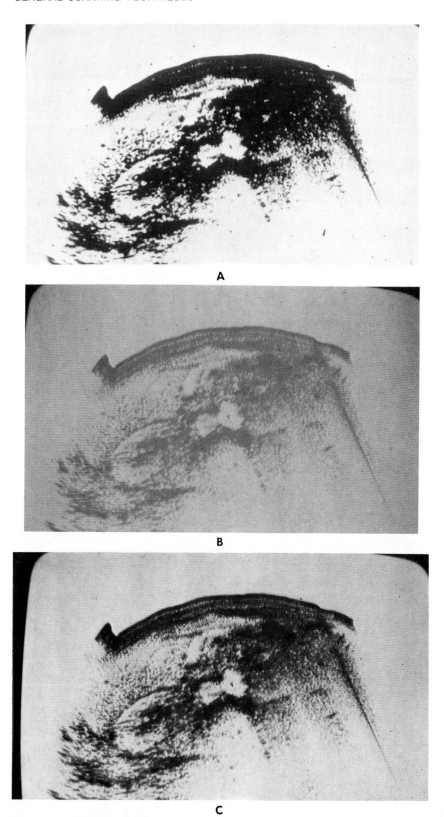

Figure 6-25. Correct setting of the monitor controls is essential if the hard copy is to look like the image on the viewing monitor.

A, A transverse abdominal scan with the contrast set too high.

B, The same picture as in *A* but with the contrast set too low.

C, The same picture as in *A* but with the contrast correctly set.

PERSPECTIVE

Now that we have learned the basics of scanning, setting the machine controls, and making good single pass scans, we are ready to be clinical ultrasonographers. The rest is window dressing. If the ultrasonographer can make a technically good scan, the picture will read itself. In the following chapters we shall discuss some practical hints which we have found useful in specific scanning situations. These are only suggestions, however, and although each ultrasonographer should try them, he should also experiment and develop the technique which works best for him.

Chapter 7

EXAMINATION OF THE ABDOMEN

We know that by this time you are eager to begin looking at patients, so we are going to start our description of specific studies with the one that is probably the most demanding—the general examination of the abdomen. Remember that it is not the purpose of this book to present pathologic findings; rather we propose to show you what constitutes a good ultrasound scan and how you go about making one. We presume that you have read and understood Chapter 6, so if you have not gone through that yet, go back and do it right now. You have read Chapter 6 already? Okay, we can go on. We shall use not only normal scans but also some pathologic ones to illustrate points related to actual ultrasound scanning; for a full description of the findings in various disease processes, however, you will have to refer to other authors (see Bibliography).

ANATOMIC LANDMARKS

At the risk of stating the obvious, it should be said at the outset that when we undertake to study any part of the body we must have a good understanding of the anatomy of the area in question so that the important landmarks there can be easily recognized. This, a fundamental principle of all ultrasound scanning, is one of the most stringent demands placed on the ultrasonographer. The understanding of cross-sectional anatomy is so important that without it the would-be ultrasonographer is lost and his efforts probably worthless. A knowledge of anatomy is important for two reasons: (1) It serves as a check on technique; that is, it lets us know whether or not the organs we want to see are visible on the scan; and (2) it allows us to relate any pathologic findings we encounter to ana-

tomic structures. The first is important because the ultrasonographer always has to ask himself if the scan is technically adequate. For example, if the examination concerns the possibility of the presence of gallstones, one must be able to say with confidence that the gallbladder is seen. The importance of the second reason is obvious: it is difficult, if not impossible, to recognize an abnormality in a structure if we do not have a good understanding of what the normal anatomy in the area is supposed to look like.

"Well, if landmarks are so important, which ones do we have to know about?" you ask. Because we almost always begin scanning the abdomen longitudinally and in the midline, let us consider longitudinal anatomy first. We begin longitudinally because we are looking for the first great anatomic landmark of the upper abdomen, the aorta (Fig. 7–1). If we are able to see the aorta in a scan made from xiphoid to several centimeters below the iliac crest, we know that we have a good acoustic window. Intestinal gas is not hiding the posterior abdominal structures, and we have a good chance of obtaining useful information about that particular abdomen.

The aorta is a satisfying structure to scan because it has nice thick walls to produce well-developed linear echoes; and the blood in its lumen transmits sound very well and is, therefore, echo-free. (In fact, the lumina of the larger blood vessels are easily seen ultrasonically. As we shall see, they are excellent anatomic locators. This visibility without the need for contrast agents is one of the truly unique features of ultrasound and is one of its greatest strengths.) As we scan down the aorta, often the wall has a "wavy" nature. This is somewhat more noticeable in young patients and is due to the pulsation of the ves-

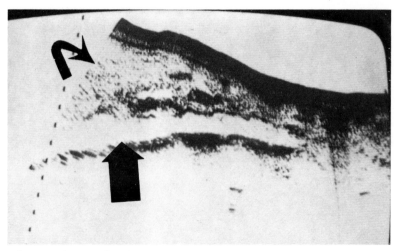

Figure 7–1. This is a longitudinal scan through the aorta (*fat arrow*) with the standard viewing orientation; that is, the patient's head is to the viewer's left. Note the wavy anterior wall of the aorta (caused by pulsations) and the wedge-shaped, relatively echo-free liver in the anterior part of the upper abdomen (*curved arrow*).

sel. Often the aorta will not lie exactly in the L,O (or midline) plane, and it will be necessary to move a centimeter or so to the left to demonstrate this vessel. Another glimpse at Figure 7–1 will show an important identifying feature of the aorta, namely, the fact that this structure tends to lie very deep high in the abdomen, under the diaphragm; but as we move toward the feet, the aorta follows the surface of the lumbar spine anteriorly and becomes somewhat smaller in diameter. We lose it at about the level of the iliac crest because it divides into the two common iliac arteries. There are several other features of this midline scan which are interesting to note: (1) The vertebral bodies are not identifiable except as a rather abrupt end of our echo information. All of the sound is reflected by the extreme mismatch in acoustical impedance between soft tissue and bone, so that, unlike the X-ray, on the ultrasound scan the bones are really not visible. (2) There is a well-defined, wedge-shaped structure anterior to the aorta in the upper abdomen. This is the liver. Note that it is homogeneously inhomogeneous (got that?), that is, it has numerous small echoes within it and is, therefore, easily recognizable as a solid organ. (We will have more to say about the liver later on.) The portion that we are seeing here is the left lobe. (3) Other vessels are easily visible either as

round or elongated, relatively small, echo-free zones anterior to the aorta. These are labeled in Figure 7–5 so that you can identify them. (These, too, will be described in greater detail below.) (4) Elsewhere, there are many nondescript echoes which are produced by bowel wall, omentum, mesentery, and other structures which cannot be named specifically.

Superficially, we see the well-defined line of the peritoneum, exterior to which there is a relatively echo-free zone, which is muscle of the anterior abdominal wall. Still further superficially, we see the subcutaneous tissue (fat), and finally the skin surface.

Now, if we move a bit to the right, say to the L+2 plane, and make another scan, we will pick up some other interesting anatomic sights, the most prominent of which is the inferior vena cava (IVC) (Fig. 7–2). This blood vessel lies next to the aorta. Although the IVC is not pulsatile its size can vary considerably. It may appear quite small; but if we ask the patient to do a Valsalva maneuver (that is, hold his breath and bear down with the abdominal muscles and diaphragm, for you who are a bit shaky on your Italian medical history of the 17th century), the IVC will get larger in diameter as the blood flow is prevented from returning to the right heart (Fig. 7–3). If you are having trouble deciding whether you

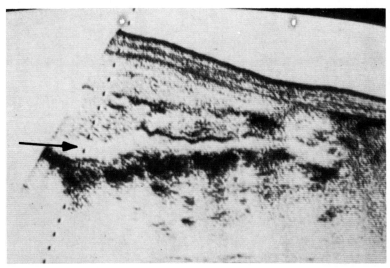

Figure 7-2. The inferior vena cava is a prominent landmark on longitudinal scans slightly to the right of midline. The IVC (*arrow*) is located just underneath the liver on this L+2 scan.

are seeing aorta or IVC, you can usually use the Valsalva maneuver to help you differentiate between the two.

Anterior to the IVC is the liver again; this time it is much thicker and occupies the entire upper abdomen. We are looking through the right lobe of the liver here. In the midst of it there are several branching linear structures which are divisions of the portal vein. We need to spend a few moments with this vessel and its tributaries because it is an important ultrasonic landmark. Let us look at Figure 7-4, which is a simplified diagram of the relationship of the splenic, superior mesenteric, and portal veins. They all lie anterior to the IVC and aorta, and the series of scans in Figure 7-5 shows the vessels as they appear in longitudinal planes, moving from just left of midline to several centimeters to its right. Once you have understood the basic arrangement, it is an easy matter to trace the vessels in a sequence of scans, just as we have in Figure 7-5; this is the best way to work out this bit of anatomy for yourself. These structures will find their way into much of what we will have to say about the abdomen, so just grit your teeth and learn to recognize them now.

You may have already noticed another interesting echo-free structure in Figure 7-5, lying slightly lower than the venous branches (that is, toward the patient's iliac crest). This, of course, is our friend, the gallbladder. We are lucky in this case be-cause the gallbladder is oriented more or less longitudinally; and, therefore, we can see it rather well in the conventional longitudinal view. We are going to look into the examination of the gallbladder in more detail below; now we want only to relate it to the other structures that we have been looking at.

If we make another scan but move out further to the right, say to L+6 (Fig. 7-6), we see that we have moved beyond most of the interesting blood vessels, but what is that posterior to the liver? You are ahead of us already; it is the right kidney (more about kidneys in Chapter 8).

Now, we want to take a look to the left of midline. We spent some time in Chapter 6 on the matter of the acoustic window, and in the upper abdomen we usually have the liver to serve as a very nice solid organ to scan through. As we move to the left, however, the liver becomes smaller; and we are much more likely to encounter gas-bearing bowel, principally the left colon and the stomach. This makes things tough. We can seldom see the left kidney from the front; and unless it is enlarged, the spleen is usually hard to demonstrate in the longitudinal scan (Fig. 7-7). A glimpse at Figure 7-8 will show what we mean; this scan made at L−3 is typical of what one gets in the left upper quadrant, and we include it here to reassure you that in anyone's hands this is an ultrasonic no man's land.

There is one more feature of the longi-

(*Text continued on p. 109.*)

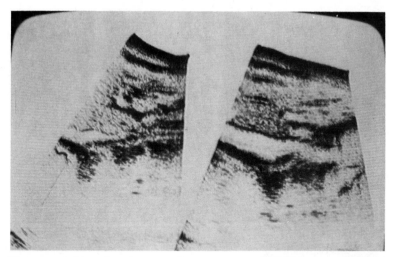

Figure 7–3. The size of the inferior vena cava can vary considerably, depending on the respiratory status of the patient: this scan was specially made to show this difference. The left half of the picture shows the IVC with the patient suspending respiration but *not* bearing down with the abdominal muscles: the IVC is not large. The right half of the picture is the same scan but the patient is bearing down (in medical jargon this is called a Valsalva maneuver) and the IVC is distended.

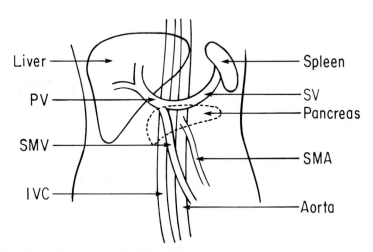

Figure 7–4. The large blood vessels of the abdomen provide excellent landmarks when scanning. This is a frontal diagrammatic representation of vessels which can be identified by the ultrasonographer. The portal venous system (PV, SMV, SV) is particularly important since the pancreas is intimately associated with these vessels. PV = portal vein, SMV = superior mesenteric vein, IVC = inferior vena cava, SV = splenic vein, SMA = superior mesenteric artery.

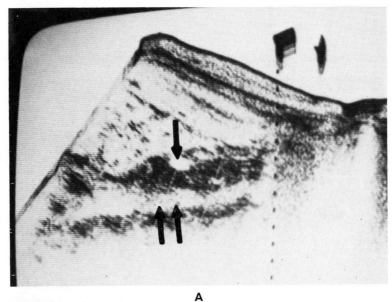

A

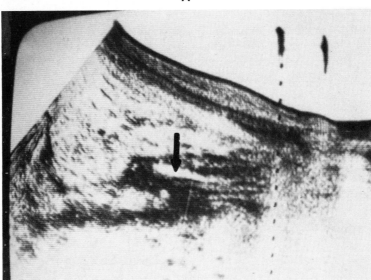

B

Figure 7–5. This is a sequence of scans made at different longitudinal locations.

A, L,O. The aorta (*double arrow*) is clearly visible to a point where it is obscured by gas in bowel. The vessel anterior to the aorta is the splenic vein (*single arrow*).

B, L+1. The aorta is no longer seen. The longitudinal vessel present is the superior mesenteric artery (*arrow*).

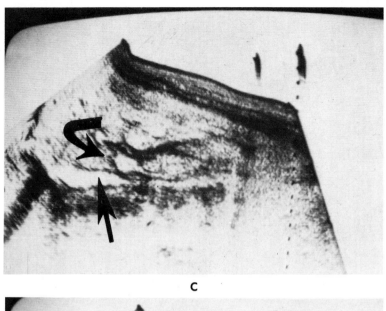

C

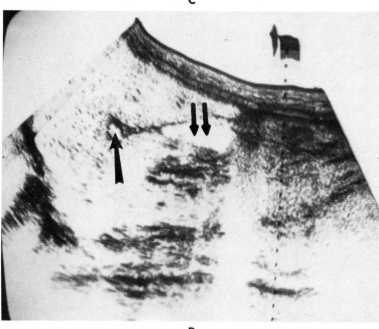

D

Figure 7–5 Continued. C, L+2. Now the inferior vena cava (*straight arrow*) has appeared. Just anterior to the IVC is a circular vessel, the portal vein (*curved arrow*).

D, L+4. The portal vein has divided, and only one branch is recognizable (*single arrow*). The gallbladder is now well seen (*double arrow*).

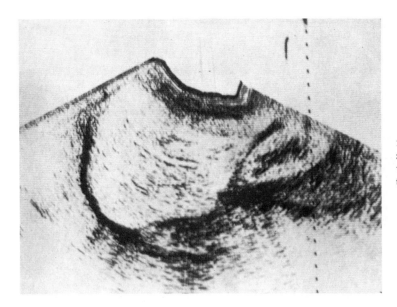

Figure 7–6. The right kidney can usually be demonstrated because of the acoustic window provided by the liver; this is an L+6 scan.

Figure 7–7. The left kidney and spleen are difficult to visualize on abdominal scans. This diagrammatic representation of an L−6 scan shows that air-containing bowel blocks our view of these organs.

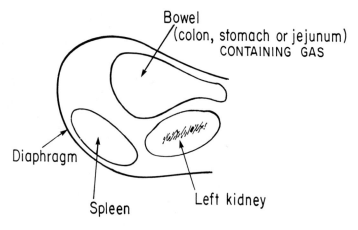

Bowel
(colon, stomach or jejunum)
CONTAINING GAS

Diaphragm

Spleen

Left kidney

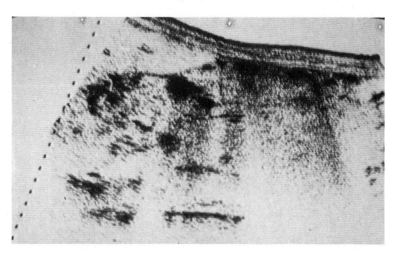

Figure 7–8. The left upper quadrant of the abdomen is the ultrasonographic no man's land: bowel, usually containing air, obscures this area. Only the left lobe of the liver can be identified on this L−3 scan.

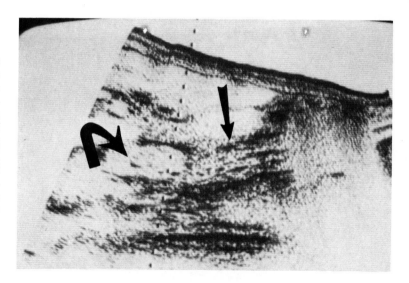

Figure 7–9. The psoas muscles can be identified on longitudinal scans a few centimeters from the midline. This is an L+3 scan and shows a small section of the upper pole of the right kidney (*curved arrow*) and the psoas muscle (*straight arrow*). It might be helpful to look at Figure 8–2 to get a better idea of these anatomic relationships.

tudinal scan which we should mention, namely, the iliopsoas muscles of the lower posterior abdominal wall. If there is little or no intestinal gas and the patient is not large, these muscles can be defined, lying between the kidney and the aorta or IVC (Fig. 7–9). But enough of this, let us move on to landmarks in the transverse views.

We will see below that it is almost always best to begin an ultrasound scan of the abdomen with some specific objective in view. Stated differently, this means that your time will be more effectively spent if you set out to examine a particular area or organ, rather than the entire abdomen. An examination of the pancreas might include only transverse scans spanning the upper abdomen from, say C+6 through C+15, for example. For the sake of laying out landmarks, however, we are going to review most of the abdomen, at least the area from the iliac crest (C0) to the level of the xiphoid (C+15 or so). As you read through this section refer to the sequence of scans in Figure 7–10.

Beginning with the lowest scan shown, in the midportion of the abdomen the aorta is clearly visible as an almost echo-free circle. The IVC is also present, again an echo-free area, somewhat oval in shape and not quite as large as the aorta. It is always surprising at first to see how far anterior the spine projects. Laterally, on either side the nondescript echoes created by bowel and other intraperitoneal structures appear, but nothing very exciting. If we move cephalad

several centimeters, things begin to pick up. Here we can see the lower portion of the right lobe of the liver (again, so obvious because of its speckled appearance), and kidneys are seen. The kidneys are separated from the spine by the psoas muscles which also appear as relatively echo-free masses. The IVC has gradually enlarged. Moving even farther toward the head, both lobes of the liver come into view, and the liver stretches across midline to the left. The gallbladder is seen as another echo-free circle nestled up under the liver edge because we are cutting across it almost at right angles to its long axis. You will note that structures to the left of midline are not defined well, and this, of course, is because of the gas in various parts of the intestinal tract (colon and stomach) which lie there and customarily contain gas. We are also able to see two smaller round echo-free areas anterior to the great vessels. The one to the patient's right is the superior mesenteric vein (SMV): to the left the superior mesenteric artery (SMA). All of these are surrounded by numerous small echoes which are produced by the pancreas and the mesentery of bowel. The normal pancreas appears as a rather dense collection of echoes lying anterior to the IVC on the right. The "head" of the pancreas is seen on the lowest sections, while the "body" and the "tail" of the gland usually lie several centimeters cephalad and stretch across midline to the left. Very often it is

(*Text continued on p. 114.*)

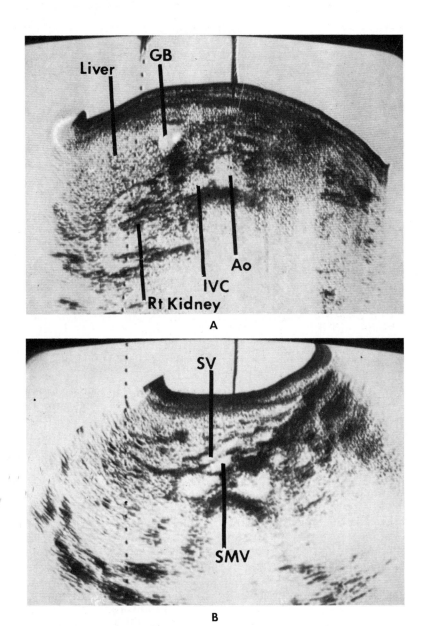

Figure 7–10. This is a sequence of scans made at different transverse levels:

A, C+2. Gas obscures the left abdomen. The aorta (Ao), inferior vena cava (IVC), right kidney, liver, and gallbladder (GB) are easily recognized.

B, C+8. We are now above the gallbladder. The left lobe of the liver is present. The splenic vein (SV) and superior mesenteric vein (SMV) are well seen.

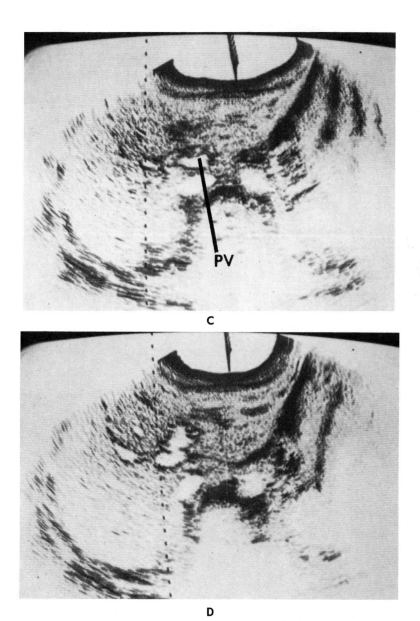

Figure 7–10 Continued. C, C+11. We are now above the right kidney. The splenic and inferior mesenteric veins have united to form the portal vein (PV). The aorta and IVC are still well visualized.

D, C+13. The branching of the portal vein within the liver is demonstrated well. Note the relative lack of echoes in the posterior portion of the right lobe of the liver.

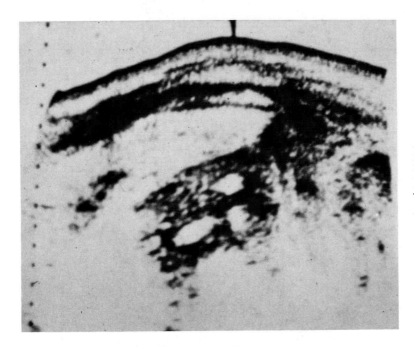

Figure 7–11. The normal pancreas can be difficult to identify. It appears as a collection of quite loud echoes just anterior to the IVC and SMV and just posterior to the liver.

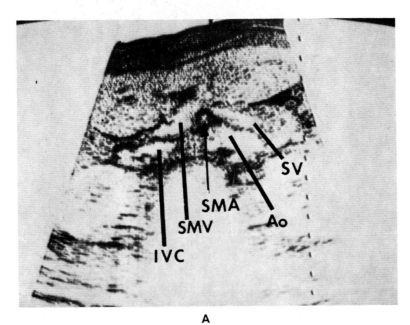

A

Figure 7–12. See legend on the opposite page.

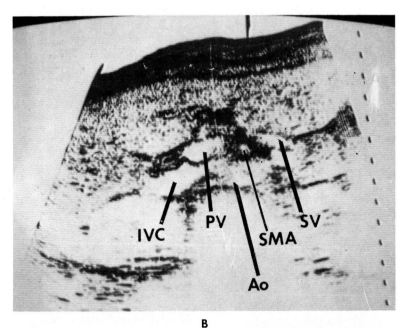

B

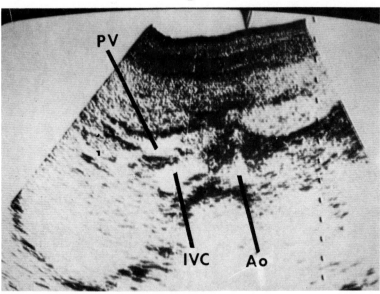

C

Figure 7–12 Continued. This sequence of transverse scans demonstrates the major vessels of the upper abdomen.

A, C+8. This scan is below the level of the confluence of the splenic vein (SV) and the superior mesenteric vein (SMV). SMA = superior mesenteric artery.

B, C+10. The portal vein (PV) is now present. The splenic vein courses cranially, a fact which explains why it is seen on both this scan and the previous one.

C, C+11. The portal vein is now branching within the liver.

hard to identify the pancreas precisely unless, of course, it is enlarged (Fig. 7–11).

The vessels in the epigastrium are important landmarks in this region, particularly for localizing the pancreas. The SMA comes off the anterior wall of the abdominal aorta and runs caudally into the mesentery of the small intestine. The SMV courses in the opposite direction from its origin in the mesentery of the small bowel to join with the splenic vein (SV) coming in from the left to form the portal vein (PV). The PV in turn enters the liver obliquely and branches there. (Check Figure 7–4 again for these relationships.) The pancreas lies anterior to all of these vessels except for the SV which generally runs along the superior or cephalic margin of the pancreas (or it may even be embedded in the upper margin of this gland). The echo pattern of the normal pancreas is so much like that of the mesentery, bowel wall, and omentum, that often we cannot identify it as a separate structure unless there is pancreatic disease. (More on this later.)

The sequence of films in Figure 7–12 demonstrates the vessels of the upper abdomen. In the middle scan we actually see both the SV and the PV near the confluence of the SV and SMV. This vessel is almost always seen and presents a nice target for the ultrasound beam. We also see that the liver has gotten quite a bit larger and now is the dominant structure present. Further cephalad we also see the PV branching within the liver. Note that the gallbladder is no longer visible. There is some controversy in ultrasound circles about whether normal (i.e., non-dilated) bile ducts can be identified and whether they can be distinguished from the portal venous radicals. We have not had much success in finding normal-sized ducts, but in those instances where the ducts are significantly dilated (because of obstruction) they can be seen ultrasonically. The biliary ducts can be identified with certainty, however, only when they can be "followed" with serial scans and connect with the gallbladder. Almost always the branching echo-free structures which one encounters in the liver are portal venous radicals; and this, too, is confirmed by "tracking" them to demonstrate that they connect with the known portal vein and its tributaries.

Once again, you will note that we have ignored the left upper quadrant. A quick glance at the series of scans will convince you that usually that region of the abdomen has little but frustration to offer the ultrasonographer. In fact, if there is an acoustic window through which to see the left upper quadrant, it should suggest that there is something wrong; the patient probably has a pathologic mass in the left upper quadrant.

SETTING THE DIALS

"That is all very good," you say, "but if I can't get the anatomy to appear on the screen, how can I tell what is is?" If you are having trouble getting pictures which look like Figure 7–5 or 7–10, you may not have your controls set properly. We will remind you only that technique is of paramount importance, and we refer you to Chapter 6 if you are having problems.

SCANNING PROBLEMS

Obviously, the scans used as illustrations so far in this chapter were obtained from ideal subjects—usually nice thin, young technologists with little fat or intestinal gas. (Like everyone who writes on ultrasound scanning, we publish only our good pictures—we do not show you our wastebasket.) The luck of the draw usually gives the beginning ultrasonographer Haystack Calhoun or some other behemoth for his first patient. This frequently provokes one or all of the following: (1) colorful cursing, (2) depression, (3) hatred of those who write books saying how simple ultrasound scanning is, (4) disillusionment with the whole ultrasound business. Do not get discouraged; remember that big patients usually make poor pictures, apparently because the interfaces presented by the adipose tissue (or very large muscles, for that matter) reflect the sound and cause deterioration of the image. In Chapter 5, where we discussed artifacts, we explained that there is nothing you can do about this (Fig. 7–13). Gas and barium in the bowel are also constant problems for us all because they rob us of an acoustic window through which to view things. If you encounter a lot of bowel gas there is nothing you or any ultrasonographer, however skilled he may be, can do about it. Fortunately, more often

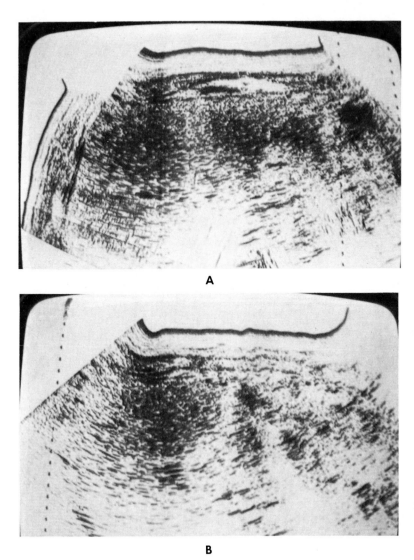

A

B

Figure 7–13. Obese patients are very difficult to scan: adipose tissue scatters and attenuates the ultrasound beam, causing poor images.
A, A C+12 scan in an obese patient.
B, An L+5 scan in the same patient. There are no recognizable anatomic structures.

than not, while we may not be able to see all the abdominal organs, and from the aesthetic standpoint the scan may be somewhat less than satisfactory, we are often able to see the area of interest and can answer the clinical question raised. Do not give up, therefore, until you have given it a good try. Finally, you will remember that in Chapter 4 we suggested that the patients fast before abdominal examinations. While this is not absolutely necessary, we must remind you that a full stomach can appear as an inhomogeneous mass in the left upper quadrant (Fig. 7–14). We do not think you need this type of hassle, so we recommend that you stick to the rules and require your patients to fast for 4 to 6 hours before you examine them.

DESIGNING THE EXAMINATION

It certainly is easier and faster to get things done if from the start we have some

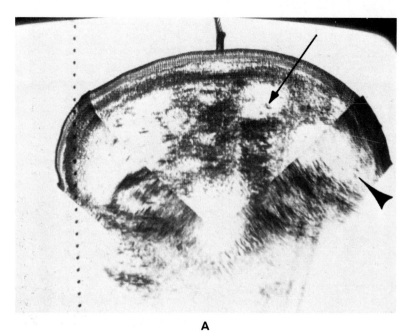

A

Figure 7–14. Food or liquid in the stomach will appear as a mass in the left upper quadrant of the abdomen.

A, A C+9 scan of a patient with an ovarian carcinoma in the left abdomen (*arrowhead*). There is a second mass adjacent to the left lobe of the liver (*arrow*); is this another tumor?

B, A C+9 scan of the same patient performed 24 hours after the scan in *A.* The tumor mass in the left abdomen is unchanged, but the second mass adjacent to the liver has been replaced by gas artifacts, suggesting that it was the stomach.

C, A C+9 CT scan performed minutes after the ultrasound scan in *B* confirms that it is the stomach which is adjacent to the liver (the patient was given intravenous and oral contrast material).

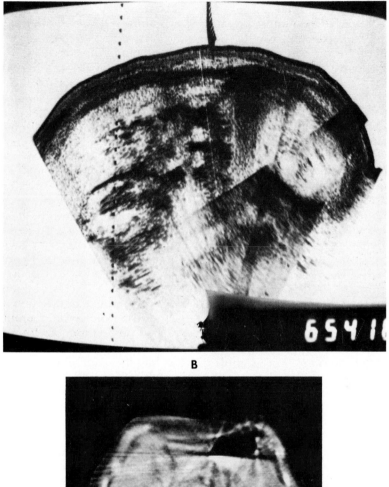

B

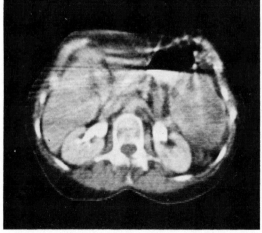

C

Figure 7–14 Continued. See legend on the opposite page.

idea about what we are looking for. Fishing expeditions waste time and are exceedingly frustrating. For this reason before we or our technologist takes transducer in hand, the clinical situation is reviewed to see what the clinician is trying to work out. This means that we have to have access to a good history. If we are examining an outpatient, the referring doctor usually has sent us a written history on the request slip, indicating clearly what the objective of the study is. (If this information is inadequate, question the patient — he often has a very good idea of what the problem is.) We go even further with in-patients and have the chart sent to the ultrasound lab with the patient, and the technologist goes through it before beginning the examination. Here, then, is another instance in which the ultrasound technologist functions as something more than a machine operator. Developing an understanding of how diseases behave symptomatically and what anatomic changes they might produce is as much a part of the ultrasonographer's training as learning to run the scanner. No need to be frightened — almost anybody can read the chart and find out what the patient's physician thinks is wrong with him, so that the ultrasound examination can be directed toward that problem. For example, if the question is one of identifying gallstones, the scanning can be limited to the gallbladder, and the time and effort spent will be considerably less than if the problem is not well defined and the entire abdomen has to be assessed.

SPECIFIC EXAMINATIONS

Aorta

The aorta is a nice place to begin when dealing with the abdomen because it is such a prominent landmark and has been the subject of ultrasonographers' attention for a long time. In almost every instance the reason for examining the aorta will be simple: confirmation or measurement of an aortic aneurysm. Judging from the literature on the subject, we seem to be a bit cavalier about aortic exams. We do not attempt to make scans at any set interval; instead we usually just begin longitudinally oriented more or less in the long axis of the

body, and scan midline and to either side, making certain that we photograph the scans that show the greatest diameter of the vessel.

When using gray scale, it is helpful to cut back the gain until there is just enough echo activity to visualize the walls. Also, it will almost always be necessary to change the angle of the transducer a bit as it is moved along the aorta because, if the beam strikes the vessel more nearly at right angles, the interface of the external wall will be more clearly seen. For example, when bringing the transducer caudally from the xiphoid, if you angle the sound beam toward the feet as you begin to see the aneurysm bulging anteriorly, the wall will be defined more clearly. As the sound beam passes over the maximum extent of the bulge, stop angling; and as you pass inferiorly, angle toward the head (Fig. 7–15).

Having recorded three or four scans longitudinally, we then switch to transverse and scan at 2 to 3 centimeter intervals over the aorta so that we can evaluate its entire length in the abdomen. Here, too, scans of interest are photographed, particularly those where the diameter is greatest; we also photograph the lowest level where the vessel is of normal caliber. If your scanner has the capability, try a few scans on bi-stable. You will find that the vessel wall is nicely seen that way, and you may want to use bi-stable to record at least the maximum bulge on every case. Do not forget to flash the centimeter marker on every scan! Also, scanning on the 2:1 scale will allow somewhat more precise measurement.

(*Heresy department:* If the patient's aorta is well calcified and you know that, there is no harm in following the aneurysm with serial lateral X-ray films of the abdomen. After all, a single X-ray is both quicker and cheaper for the patient and has the advantage that almost any physician can interpret it.)

In scanning the aorta, bowel artifacts are usually not so important because the walls of this great vessel can be easily seen. (Another hint: if you have trouble finding the aorta on longitudinal scans, try a few transverse ones. Often the vessel can be seen only through a small window, not easily found longitudinally.) If you have the gain set properly, you may be able to see clot within an aneurysm. In general, it

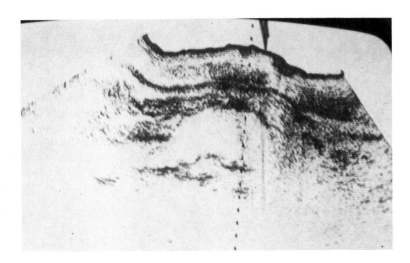

Figure 7–15. Most aortic aneurysms are easy to demonstrate; but when the aorta is tortuous, it can be difficult to show the walls clearly. In this situation it is helpful to decrease the gain until the aortic walls are well defined and to try to keep the sound beam perpendicular to the aorta as much as possible. Single pass scanning is not important in this case since the aortic walls are specular reflectors and gray scale is not necessary.

is the external dimension of the vessel that we are interested in and which ultrasound displays so well.

Retroperitoneum

It seems only sensible to say a thing or two about the retroperitoneum at this point, because scanning this area is intimately linked to the aorta. We are usually looking for enlarged lymph nodes and there is no real trick to this; the technique is almost the same as for the aorta. Frequently, however, lymphadenopathy will extend into the pelvis along the sacrum; and, therefore, the longitudinal scans should be carried further caudally. This, of course, presents problems because the bowel in the lower abdomen almost always has gas in it so that the pre-sacral area may not be seen well. Fortunately, disease of the retroperitoneum other than lymphadenopathy (for example, hematoma or abscess) is easy to recognize because it produces lesions which are usually more nearly echo-free, are focal rather than generalized, and are often of sufficient size that the bowel is pushed out of the way. Lymphadenopathy is almost always found anterior

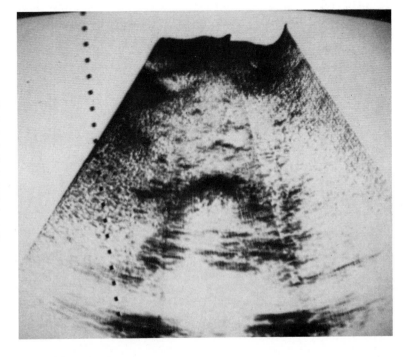

Figure 7–16. When the lymph nodes near the spine and aorta are involved with tumor they enlarge and encircle the aorta, giving a "doughnut" appearance. Pathologic lymph nodes produce very few echoes and usually stand out quite clearly from their surroundings. This patient had a metastatic testicular tumor.

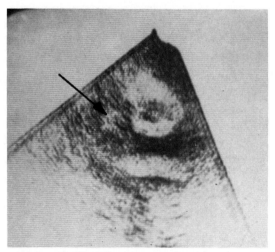

Figure 7–17. The normal adrenals take considerable patience in scanning. It may be necessary to try many different positions. One of the most useful is with the patient lying on his side. This scan of the normal left adrenal gland (*arrow*) was made with the patient lying on his right side; the scanning plane was longitudinal and passed through the upper pole of the left kidney and the aorta.

to and alongside the aorta and IVC, and the nodes are always relatively echo-free and rather easily differentiated from their surrounding tissue (Fig. 7–16). As with any abdominal scan, it is helpful to evaluate the retroperitoneum both longitudinally and transversely, particularly if an abnormality is suspected because of findings on a scan or if there is difficulty in seeing the retroperitoneum longitudinally because of gas.

The adrenals are important retroperitoneal structures which should not be forgotten. They are hard to see when scanned

posteriorly because of overlying ribs. When scanned from the front, however, at least the right adrenal can sometimes be seen, especially if it is enlarged. Here, too, a pathologic process is very likely to be relatively echo-free; and this tends to aid us in recognizing any abnormality which might be present. In the case of the adrenal the longitudinal scan is the really important one, and differentiation between a mass in the upper pole of the kidney and one in the adrenal is very important. If the adrenal area cannot be seen from the front, turning the patient prone or on his side may help (Fig. 7–17). In general, however, it is not useful to look at the retroperitoneum, except for the kidney and adrenal, with the patient lying prone.

Gallbladder

Ultrasound has proven to be a big help in the evaluation of gallbladder disease, particularly in the identification of gallstones. Much of the early difficulty with this examination arose from problems with technique, and the development of gray scale has made it considerably easier to examine this organ. Here again, it is helpful to have an X-ray study to look at, because we want to scan the gallbladder longitudinally in its longest axis. If a cholecystogram is not available, however, all is not lost; all you need do is turn your scanning head so that you can scan in a plane roughly parallel to the right costal margin, ask the patient to take a deep breath and hold it, and make a survey scan (Fig. 7–18). There is fre-

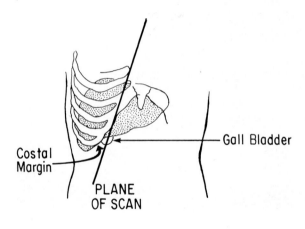

Costal Margin

PLANE OF SCAN

Gall Bladder

Figure 7–18. It takes a few trial scans to find the axis of the gallbladder. Usually it is near the costal margin. Longitudinal scans of the gallbladder should all be made parallel to its axis.

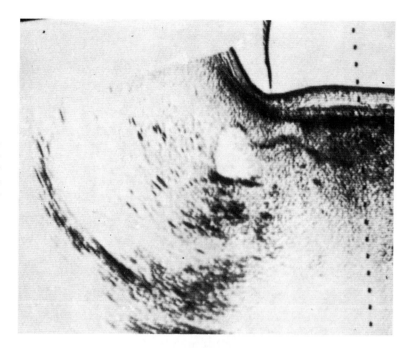

Figure 7–19. A single pass scan is best for visualizing the gallbladder. It may be necessary to angle the transducer sharply to stay over an acoustic window.

quently gas in the hepatic flexure of the colon or the duodenal bulb, so the liver must be used as an acoustic window. In this examination, more than anywhere else in the abdomen, having the patient suspend respiration in deep inspiration is vitally important. You will have to explore around a bit, moving up and down parallel to the costal margin until the gallbladder comes into view. Once you have caught it, you may well have to alter the angle with respect to the long axis of the body to bring the plane of your scan into the long axis of the gallbladder. The scanning motion is a clean sweep, the lower portion of which is sectored (Fig. 7–19).

It is very important to scan in multiple planes parallel to the axis of the gallbladder so as to avoid overlooking any area where stones might lie (Fig. 7–20). It is equally important to use a little imagination in locating the gallbladder. This is one organ which does vary in position with respect to body build. It will be nearly horizontal in a short, squat patient and almost vertical in a tall, skinny one. The more nearly vertical it is, the easier it will be for you to visualize. We do not bother to indicate coordinates when examining the gallbladder. The angulation necessary to visualize this viscus in its long axis will have to be determined during the study

anyway; and once the gallbladder is seen in its long axis, movement a centimeter or two to the right or left will soon put the beam outside of the organ.

We rely on the demonstration of the echo-free lumen to recognize the gallbladder. Sometimes, when the gallbladder is contracted because it is diseased and con-

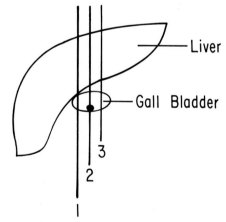

Figure 7–20. Small gallstones can be missed unless scans are made every 5 mm. This is a diagrammatic cross-section of a gallbladder containing a small stone. Planes 1, 2, and 3 are possible longitudinal scanning planes. Only plane 2 would demonstrate the gallstone; the gallbladder would appear normal at planes 1 and 3.

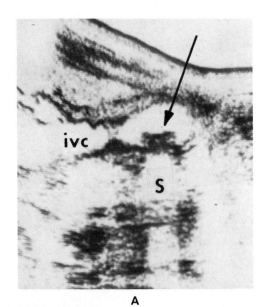

A

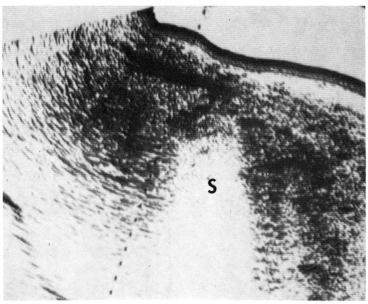

B

Figure 7–21. Gallstones can be recognized either by the echoes they produce within the gallbladder or by the ultrasonic "shadow" they cast.

A, The "classic" appearance of gallstones: the stones produce echoes within the gallbladder lumen *(arrow)* and cast an ultrasonic shadow (S). A portion of the inferior vena cava (ivc) is seen because this scan was made obliquely, 2 centimeters below the right costal margin.

B, When the gallbladder is completely filled with stones, only the ultrasonic shadow betrays their existence (S).

tains stones, the lumen is not visible. All would be lost for the ultrasonographer if it were not for the fact that gallstones frequently reflect all of the sound, and therefore, cast a well-defined acoustic shadow (Fig. 7–21). Remember, however, that bowel gas also casts an acoustic shadow of sorts, so we have to guard against mistaking gas in duodenum or colon for a shrunken gallbladder containing stones. It often helps in this situation to scan transversely. (Be sure to mark the location of this suspicious shadow on the patient's skin so that you will know when you are scanning over

it in the new plane.) Scanning transversely, the goal is to try to decide whether or not the shadow is arising from a site compatible with the position of the gallbladder. Sometimes it is even possible to recognize the gallbladder lumen, not seen on longitudinal scans (Fig. 7–22).

We want to emphasize here the importance of having the patient fasting or NPO for 10 to 12 hours before the gallbladder is scanned. The reason for this is obvious: we have a much better chance of identifying the gallbladder if it is filled with bile. By the same token, if the scan is done in con-

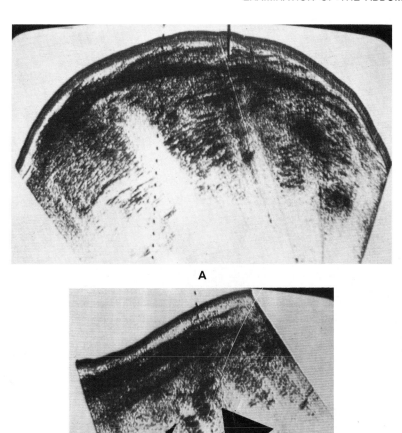

A

B

Figure 7-22. Transverse scans of the gallbladder are often helpful in separating a shadow cast by a gallstone from one cast by bowel gas.

A, A true "shadow sign" from gallstones. The shadow arises from the expected location of the gallbladder.

B, A false "shadow sign" from bowel gas *(fat arrow)*: although the shadow is arising from a location compatible with the gallbladder, the presence of the small, contracted, real gallbladder *(wavy arrow)* shows us that the shadow is being cast by bowel.

junction with an oral cholecystogram, it is important to scan the patient *before* a fatty meal is given. This brings us to a description of how we fit the ultrasound scan of the gallbladder into our work-up of gallbladder disease. We do not believe that ultrasound should be used as a substitute for the oral cholecystogram. We scan the gallbladder with ultrasound only if it is not visualized adequately on a single oral dose of contrast agent, or if there is a question raised by the oral study about the possible presence of stones. If we can demonstrate stones satisfactorily on an ultrasound scan,

no further radiologic work-up is indicated in most instances. Also, in the case of a patient suspected of having acute cholecystitis, a scan of the gallbladder should be done before an oral or intravenous examination. If stones are present, the ultrasound will almost certainly demonstrate them. This, together with appropriate history, physical findings, and laboratory abnormalities, will confirm the diagnosis.

The recognition of gallstones ultrasonically is generally not difficult because they so often produce an acoustic shadow, as described above. Bear in mind, however,

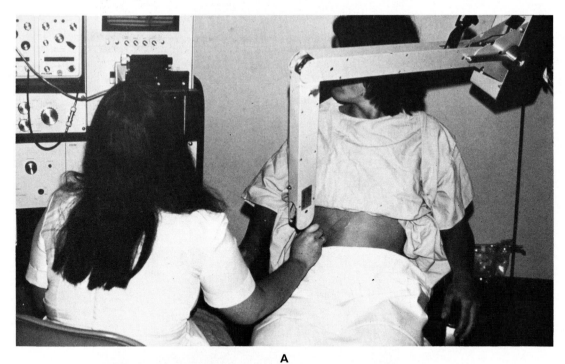

A

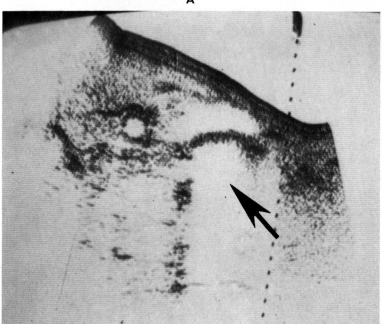

B

Figure 7–23. Scanning the gallbladder with the patient upright can often help resolve a question of gallstones.

A, An upright scan is easily accomplished by having the patient sit in a chair and bringing the scanning arm over the left shoulder.

B, Is this large shadow *(arrow)* due to a layer of gallstones on the bottom of the gallbladder or is it arising from air-containing bowel just underneath the gallbladder?

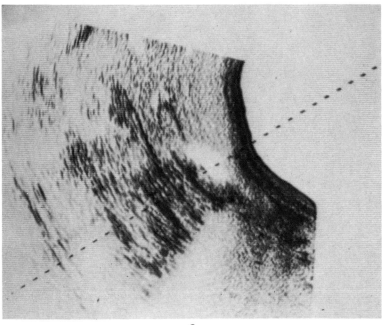

C

Figure 7–23 Continued. C, The same gallbladder as in B, scanned in the upright position; small stones and their shadow have shifted position, confirming the diagnosis.

that you are at liberty to manipulate the patient's position to help confirm your suspicions. The simple maneuver of scanning the patient while he is seated often will show that the stones suspected on the recumbent examination have shifted with gravity (Fig. 7–23).

A final word: if gallstones are found, it is probably good practice to sneak a look at the pancreas because of the association of pancreatitis (recognized ultrasonically by enlargement of the gland) and the passage of a gallstone. It may, in fact, be the pancreatic trouble which is giving the patient his bellyache, and the documentation of pancreatic edema will be most helpful to the clinician.

Liver

The liver is a nice organ to study ultrasonically because it is large and much of it can be seen well. The problem in this area, however, is the ribs. That part of the liver above the costal margin is difficult to scan; but here again, a deep inspiration can help to increase what we can see. Moreover, much of the liver is quite close to the end of the transducer, so this means that it may be necessary to vary TGC or gain or to change to a higher transducer frequency

(with shorter focus) to bring the relatively near field into clear view. No matter what we do, it is often very hard to achieve uniform echo activity throughout the liver—especially if it is cirrhotic and produces numerous very strong echoes. Often it is impossible to see deep into the lateral aspect of the right lobe or high up beneath the diaphragm. Even in the normal patient, these areas tend to be relatively echo-free; and if this is not appreciated, the finding can easily be misinterpreted as a relatively echo-free lesion—abscess or tumor, for example (Fig. 7–24).

Sectoring is generally the most reliable way to produce scans when the liver parenchyma itself is the area of interest; and in transverse scans between the costal margins or when there is the need to look between the ribs, it is the only way to produce a suitable picture (Fig. 7–25). In longitudinal scans, sectoring produces good images also, so we use it there as well.

There is one further anatomic point of some importance: a portion of the liver, the caudate lobe (Fig. 7–26), can be easily mistaken for the head of the pancreas if the patient is scanned only transversely. If a longitudinal scan is done in addition, however, it is almost always possible to see that the structure in question is a part of the

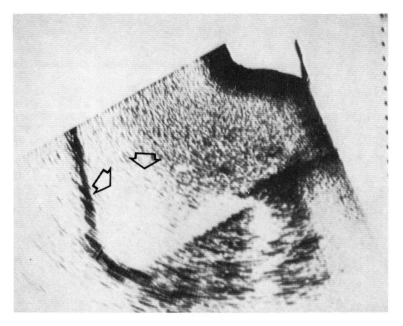

Figure 7–24. There is often an echoless area deep in the right lobe of the liver on longitudinal scans. This is an L+6 scan of a normal liver showing such a region (*open arrows*). This area, which arises when attenuation of the sound beam is greater than the capacity of the TCG, must not be mistaken for a pathologic lesion.

liver. There is also a rather infamous loud echo which frequently appears in the liver near the junction of the right and left lobes on transverse scans (Fig. 7–27). The cause of this "liver echo" is not clear; but it is relatively common; and, therefore, we mention it so that you will not be misled when you encounter it.

What are our objectives in scanning the liver? First, we can assess the overall size of the organ easily and quickly. (We offer no standard measurements here, but with a bit of experience, you will know what to expect regarding liver size.) Second, the hepatic texture is easily evaluated. Some generalized liver diseases produce a striking change in echo activity. Cirrhosis, for example, greatly increases the number and the strength of echoes produced by the liver parenchyma, and this is easily noted (Fig. 7–28). So far it has not been possible to distinguish specific hepatic diseases (cirrhosis and certain types of hepatitis tend to look very much the same), but the normal and abnormal livers do differ in appearance. Back to our objectives: focal lesions such as metastases can be identified readily if they are located in regions accessible to

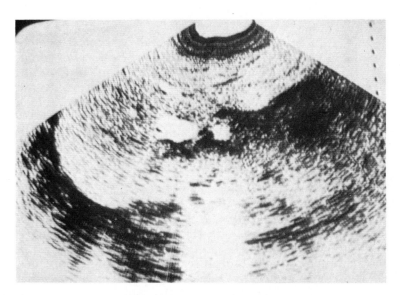

Figure 7–25. It is very important that the sound beam not pass through any bowel or ribs if the liver parenchyma is to be evaluated.

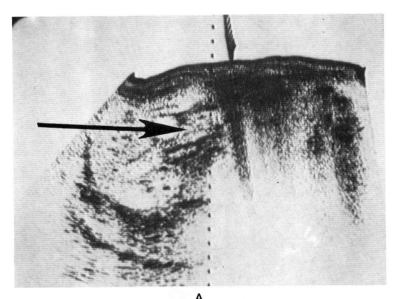

A

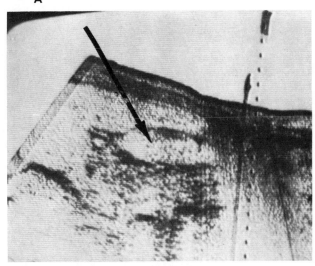

B

Figure 7–26. The caudate lobe of the liver can sometimes mimic a mass in the head of the pancreas.

A, A C+10 scan showing a prominent— but normal—caudate lobe (*arrow*).

B, An L+2 scan of the same patient as in A, again showing the large caudate lobe.

the transducer. You will find that metastases may produce either more, less, or the same number and strength of echoes as normal liver. The problems here, of course, are the fact that there are too many false negative examinations for ultrasound to serve as an effective screening procedure for metastasis, and much of the liver is hidden by ribs. Finally, there is the question of dilated bile ducts. Differentiation between big ducts and portal venous radicals is difficult and in many cases impossible, as we have said previously. When extrahepatic biliary obstruction is present, however, there are usually other observations, such as a big gallbladder, gallstones, or pancrea-

tic mass, to support laboratory data of obstruction. Remember, we are not working in a vacuum; it is always best to use all the data available.

Pancreas

One of the most important attributes of ultrasound when used in the abdomen has proved to be the ease with which it can display pancreatic disease—provided, of course, that the pancreas is not hidden by bowel gas. Because of the relationship of the pancreas to the major epigastric vessels, it is easiest to begin scanning trans-

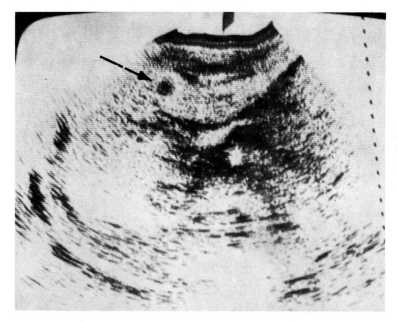

Figure 7–27. There is a loud echo *(arrow)* which appears near the junction of the right and left lobes of the liver on high transverse scans such as this C+15. This echo, probably originating from the ligamentum teres, is *normal* — it is present in almost three-quarters of our patients.

versely. As we stated above, a normal pancreas cannot always be clearly identified because it produces very dark echoes which are very similar to the structures in its vicinity. The key to the identification of the pancreas is locating the splenic vein, which almost always runs along the upper margin of the pancreas. The pancreas itself stretches obliquely across the posterior abdominal wall from about the level of the hilum of the right kidney to the hilum of the spleen in the left upper quadrant. If the splenic vein is not along the margin of the pancreas, it lies just posterior to its superior or cephalad portion. It stands to reason, then, that the pancreas will be found a centimeter or two caudad to the splenic vein on either transverse or longitudinal scans.

We believe that it is always easier to assess the pancreas transversely, and we do

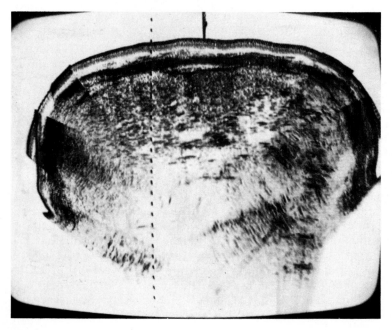

Figure 7–28. Diffuse liver disease such as cirrhosis causes the liver parenchyma to produce many loud echoes. Such livers appear very black on the monitor and attenuate the sound beam so much that it may be impossible to scan through them. This is a C+12 scan of a cirrhotic patient.

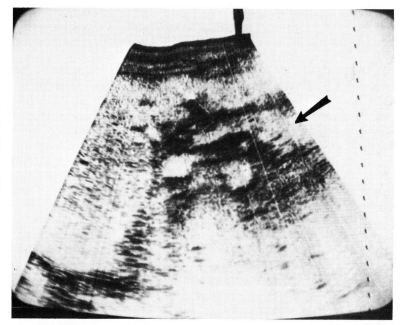

Figure 7–29. Any pathologic process tends to enlarge the pancreas and make it more echo-free and thus easier to see. This C+11 section shows a small mass in the body of the pancreas (*arrow*), which was a pancreatic neoplasm.

this by locating the splenic vein and then scanning in planes 1, 2, or 3 centimeters toward the patient's feet. With careful gray scale technique it may be possible to see the normal pancreas. We do not routinely scan the pancreas obliquely. This is recommended in the literature, but in our experience has not proved to be necessary or particularly helpful. Almost any gross pathologic process which affects the pancreas — tumor, edema from pancreatitis, or cyst — will enlarge it and decrease its echo production (Figs. 7–29 and 7–30). A mass with fewer echoes than normal lying anterior to the superior mesenteric vein, the superior mesenteric artery, or the IVC and below the level of the splenic vein is likely to be pancreatic in origin.

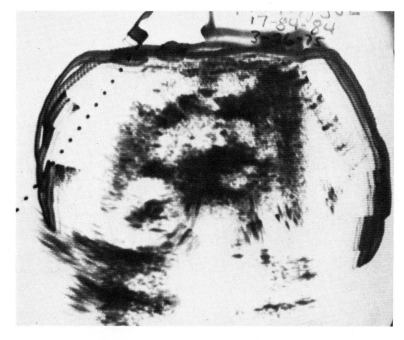

Figure 7–30. Pancreatitis makes the entire pancreas edematous and echoless, causing it to stand out dramatically from its surroundings.

Having done the transverse scans, we switch to longitudinal position and scan again from left of aorta to right of IVC. Any bona fide mass will be readily seen on both longitudinal and transverse scans and, if pancreatic in origin, will lie caudad to the splenic vein. The region of the tail of the pancreas presents a special problem area, because of the probability that the left upper quadrant will be obscured by gas. There is really nothing that can be done about this. Again, experience shows that while the tail of the pancreas might not be visible if normal, when involved by a pathologic process, it is usually enlarged and can, therefore, be seen (probably because gas-bearing bowel is displaced).

Several maneuvers have been suggested as a means of improving things in the left upper quadrant so that the tail of the pancreas can be seen more reliably. The first of these is scanning the patient prone. This technique can be helpful, especially if the patient is thin. It is cumbersome, however, and will not endear you to the patient if his belly is sore. When the patient is very large or muscular, scanning from the back will be of no real help. Others have tried filling the stomach with water or a water-filled balloon. We mention this only to condemn it; we have tried these maneuvers, find them of no real benefit, and do not use

them. Simethicone by mouth has been recommended to decrease bowel gas. We have no experience with this, but judge from what is written that it, too, is not helpful. A bowel prep, that is, laxatives coupled with low residue diet, has been suggested by some and can be useful. This greatly complicates preparation, however, and is probably more trouble than it is worth. If the patient is to have a bowel prep for another purpose, for example, an intravenous urogram or barium enema, it is worth your while to try to take advantage of this in scheduling the ultrasound scan. Finally, it might help to be able to scan the standing patient, although with most present ultrasound machines this is difficult or impossible to do and is, therefore, impractical for most ultrasonographers.

Brief mention should be made of the potential error of mistaking the stomach or the colon for a mass in the tail of the pancreas. When this problem arises, it is usually the stomach which is the source of difficulty, and a question or two directed at finding when the patient last took something by mouth will help you decide whether or not you will profit by scanning him again after a short wait to allow the stomach to empty (Fig. 7–14). Often we scan the patient on a second day if we have doubts about masses found in the tail of the

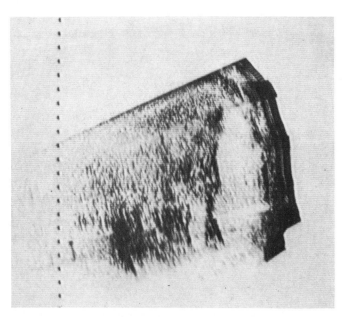

Figure 7–31. The normal-sized spleen is difficult to visualize in the supine position; sometimes portions of it can be seen between ribs, well down in the left flank. If examination of the spleen has been specifically requested, the patient should be scanned in the right lateral decubitus and prone positions.

pancreas; if such a mass is present the second time around, there is a much greater chance of its being truly pathologic.

A final word about the pancreas: you will see that we have not advanced any measurements for the normal pancreas. We have found none that are useful in everyday work and believe that here, too, experience will allow you to decide what is normal. The rule of thumb which says that if the pancreas is easily recognized, it must be abnormal may be a bit extreme, but for most ultrasonographers it is a fairly reasonable statement.

Spleen

Of all abdominal organs the spleen has received the least attention from the ultrasound world, and that is simply because it is hidden way up there under the ribs. It is no big item, however, to visualize the spleen (especially if it is enlarged and extends down below the costal margin); how-

ever, the normal spleen can be elusive. One way to solve this is to roll the patient onto his right side so that you can get around back to get at the spleen through the posterior ribs. We usually just scan the patient supine, however, in suspended inspiration. We scan transversely, running the transducer between the ribs—usually between 10 and 11 laterally; and we use a 3.5 MHz, 13 mm diameter transducer with medium internal focus for this because it is small and will usually fit between the ribs (Fig. 7–31). The spleen is monotonously homogeneous with many weak (light gray) echoes; and it usually has a nice smooth surface (actually the spleen is just a sac of blood). If you have trouble seeing it, it is unlikely to be abnormal.

Before we leave the abdomen, let us urge you to use your imagination and ingenuity when scanning. We offer you the basic moves in this game; as all of us know, how-to manuals are just for getting started. The real fun is in seeing where you can take it from there.

Chapter 8

EXAMINATION OF THE KIDNEY

In many ways the kidneys are among the most satisfying organs to evaluate ultrasonically; they can usually be seen well, and gas and patient size usually do not interfere seriously with the examination. Renal problems do, however, demand expertise in performance of the examination, so we will describe a routine that will enable you to whip off an examination of the kidneys rapidly with confidence in your results. As in all aspects of B-scanning, experience makes evaluation of the kidneys go much more smoothly; so do not despair if your first attempts are less than exciting. The demonstration of a renal cyst is certainly a satisfying experience, well worth striving for.

RENAL ANATOMY

Let us first take a look at the anatomy of the kidneys and their environs, because this influences very much the way we go about studying them. The kidneys lie in what is called the retroperitoneum; that is, they lie *in* the posterior wall of the abdomen, excluded from the intra-abdominal structures such as liver, spleen, and the intestines by the lining of the abdominal cavity, the peritoneum (Fig. 8–1). The kidneys are nestled in a bed of fat, which serves to cushion them a bit; and viewed from the front, they and their bed of fat lie on the big muscles of the back. They are oriented more or less up and down; that is, their longest dimension parallels the spinal column. They are angled somewhat so that their lower poles are not only farther from the spine than the upper, but are also more anterior. The kidneys lie along the iliopsoas muscle; and, if you recall what they look like on a plain film of the abdomen,

you will have a good idea of the relationship of the kidneys to the psoas muscles and the spinal column (Fig. 8–2).

SCANNING POSITIONS

We can see that the kidneys sit much closer to the skin of the back than to the anterior abdominal wall. Moreover, there is nothing but several layers of muscle, some fat, and skin between the transducer and the kidneys when we examine the patient from behind. One advantage of scanning from behind, therefore, is that we have a good acoustic window; and intestinal gas does not get in the way. Occasionally, however, the upper pole lies under the lower ribs, limiting our view of the kidneys. One further point in terms of position of the kidneys: usually the left lies a bit higher than the right. (It is more accurate to say that the kidney on the side *opposite the liver* is the higher.) This means that the upper pole of the left kidney is more likely to be hidden by a rib than the right.

Bearing all of this in mind, then, we find it easiest to do renal examinations with the patient prone, lying with a pillow under the abdomen to flex the lumbar spine so that the lower ribs are moved toward the head slightly to give a better view of the kidneys. (Fig. 8–3). Sometimes, we will be asked to look at the kidneys of a patient with a painful abdomen. In such cases it may not be possible to turn the patient onto his belly. We have been able to get around this problem by having the patient lie on his side, usually turned more or less prone. We then scan the uppermost kidney from the back.

Occasionally, it is best to examine the right kidney with the patient supine, using the right lobe of the liver as an acoustic

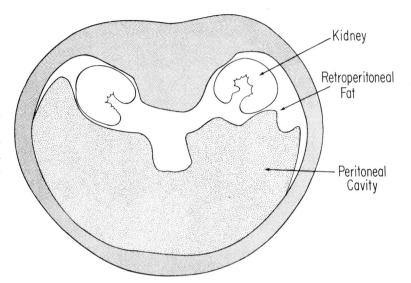

Figure 8–1. The kidneys are retroperitoneal organs surrounded by fat. It is usually easier to scan them via the back muscles rather than through the bowel.

window. Unfortunately, this trick almost never works with the left kidney because there is no acoustic window, only intestinal gas, in the left upper quadrant of the abdomen. Although we believe it best to approach the kidneys posteriorly, you should be imaginative enough to deviate from convention to get around an obstacle which would otherwise prevent a satisfactory examination.

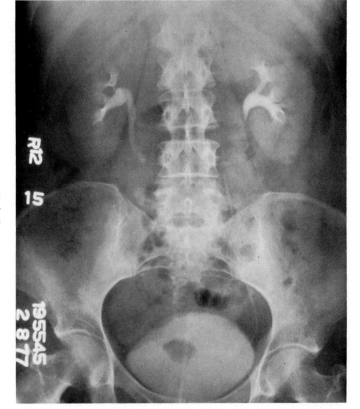

Figure 8–2. The kidneys lie at an angle to the long axis of the patient. This X-ray film from an intravenous pyelogram shows the axis of the kidneys and their relationship to the spine and psoas muscles.

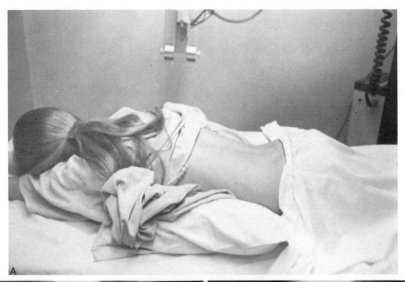

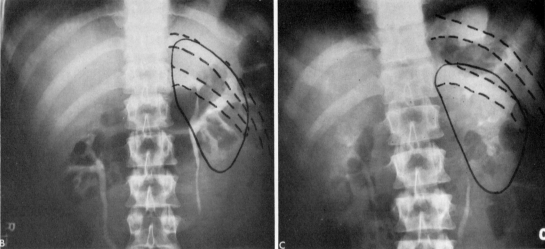

Figure 8–3. Flexing the spine by having the patient lie prone on a pillow helps bring the kidneys out from underneath the ribs.

A, The patient in position for a renal scan.

B, An X-ray film of the kidneys taken with the patient supine: notice how the eleventh and twelfth ribs cover the upper pole of the left kidney.

C, The same patient as in B, but the radiograph was taken with the patient in the position shown in A: The ribs no longer cover as much of the kidney.

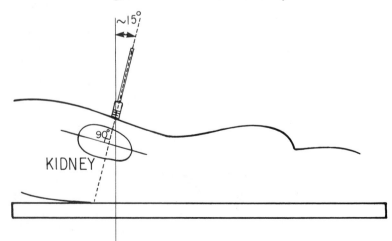

Figure 8–4. Transverse scans of the kidney should be performed at right angles to the renal axis. This usually involves angling the scanning head 15 to 20° toward the patient's head.

SCANNING PLANES

We begin the examination with transverse scans. The patient must suspend respiration; but the question of what phase of respiration to use (inspiration, expiration, or midway between the two) has to be decided in each case, depending upon the relationship of the kidneys to the ribs and the iliac crest. Usually maximum inspiration is best because this pushes the upper poles of the kidneys down to the point where they are below the ribs. Again, flexibility is necessary; and if the kidney is more easily seen on expiration, we use that. Remember that the same phase of respiration should be used throughout the examination.

For the transverse scans the scanner head should be angled slightly so that the scan is made in a plane roughly perpendicular to the long axis of the kidney, as shown in Figure 8–4. It is difficult to be precise about this until you have done a longitudinal scan to see how the long axis actually lies, but it is easy enough to guess at it; and usually angling the ultrasound beam 10 to 15 degrees toward the head will do the trick. Three or four transverse scans are done at various levels along the kidney. At each level, the middle of the kidney is indicated on the skin by making a dot with marking solution, as shown in Figure 8–5. This will define the long axis of the kidney for longitudinal scanning. As few as three transverse scans may be enough—one through both upper and lower poles, a third through the middle of the kidney. If any abnormalities are encountered, more scans are often made. It is important to be certain that no part of the kidney is overlooked.

Once the transverse sections have been made, the long axis of the kidney is laid out by a line connecting the marks placed on the skin of the back. The scanning head is rotated and the longitudinal scans are made parallel to the line marked on the back. Again, it may be necessary to angle the scanning head; we try to keep the transducer more or less perpendicular to the skin of the back. A second series of scans is then made—three or four perhaps—at 1 centimeter intervals, covering the kidney from medial to lateral. If an abnormality is encountered, more scans may well be needed.

We usually examine each kidney individually, transversely as well as longitudinally. If we are asked to look at one kidney only, we do not necessarily study the opposite one, particularly if the kidney is normal. We seldom attempt to include both kidneys on a single transverse scan. The exception here might be for the sake of illustrating a finding present on one side only, but including on the same scan a view of the normal opposite kidney.

COORDINATES

As we mentioned in Chapter 6, we use a modified coordinate system for renal scans, because longitudinal sections are usually obtained at an angle to the midsagittal plane and thus cannot be readily identified with our regular coordinate system. *Transverse* sections are labeled using the standard "C±X" system where "X" represents the displacement of the scan plane in centimeters from the line connecting the iliac crests. Sections toward the head are positive, and toward the feet negative. We omit the angulation of the scan plane since this is understood to be whatever angle is perpendicular to the axis of the kidney (usually about 10 to 15 degrees). *Longitudinal* sections are labeled as "L±X"; however, the "X" no longer refers to the displacement of the scan from the midsagittal line. Instead, it describes the relationship of the scan to the *axis line of the kidney*. Displacements toward the patient's right side are considered positive, and those toward the patient's left side negative. A scan bearing the legend "L–2" was, therefore, performed 2 centimeters to the left of the line drawn down the long axis of the kidney. (Remember this is the *patient's* left.) Of course, we must also label the scan "Right" or "Left" corresponding to which kidney we are scanning, so that a complete designation would go something like this: "LEFT, L–2," meaning left kidney, longitudinal scan in a plane 2 centimeters to the patient's left of the axis line of the kidney (Fig. 8–5).

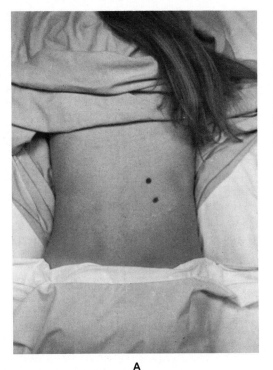

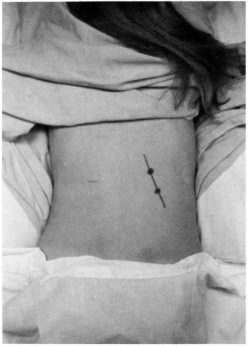

A

B

C

Figure 8–5. Longitudinal renal scans should be made parallel to the long axis of the kidney.

A, The renal axis is located by making two or more transverse scans and marking the center point of the kidney on the patient's skin.

B, A line drawn through these points defines the long axis of the kidney.

C, Longitudinal scans are labeled according to their displacement from this renal axis. In the case illustrated here the scan would be labeled "L–2," meaning "longitudinal section 2 centimeters to the left (*patient's left*) of the renal axis." The picture must also be labeled "right" or "left" corresponding to the kidney being scanned.

AXIS DRAWN THRU MID POINT SKIN MARKS

PLANE OF SCAN 2 cm LEFT OF AXIS DESIGNATED "RIGHT, L-2"

HARDWARE CONSIDERATIONS

We cannot agree on the best scale to use for renal examinations; one of us insists on the 3:1 scale, while the other prefers 2:1. It seems reasonable to use the scale you feel most comfortable with. Certainly, any image smaller than 3:1 will probably cause you to lose valuable information; and kidneys above infant size often will be too large for the 1:1 scale. We avoid, as always, the "zoom." In general, we believe that enlarging the image with the "zoom" degrades the picture (except when scanning on the 1:1 scale). If enlargement does seem advantageous, it is almost always better to change to a larger scale, i.e., from 3:1 to 2:1. (For purposes of teaching or special demonstration, enlarging the image with the "zoom" is sometimes a useful trick, but it almost never aids in diagnosis.)

We begin scanning with the 2.25 MHz, 19 mm diameter transducer with long internal focus, because this gives good definition at the depth at which both kidneys lie in the adult. If the patient is small (i.e., a thin adult or child), we may use a 3.5 MHz, 13 mm diameter transducer with a medium internal focus. For newborns and young infants the 5 MHz, 6 mm diameter transducer with short internal focus is used; and usually we scan on the 1:1 scale when using this high frequency.

Setting the dials is not difficult and is not different from ordinary abdominal scanning. The gain should be set so that there is adequate echo information without serious interference from reverberation artifact. How do you tell when enough is enough? We find that with gray scale scanners the renal parenchyma is usually light gray and that the central or hilar structures are well defined by a strong black echo. The subcutaneous and other perirenal tissues usually show up as medium to very dark echoes, demonstrated as short lines paralleling the transducer/skin interface. Figure 8–6 shows a kidney at appropriate gain setting. If the gain is too low (Fig. 8–7), both peri- and intrarenal echoes will begin to fade, especially the echoes beneath or anterior to the kidney. Consequently, there will be loss of its anterior surface, and renal parenchymal lesions may be missed. On the other hand, if the setting is too high (Fig. 8–8), reverberation will begin to obscure the kidneys; the parenchyma will begin to lose its "clean" appearance, and there will be "echoes" in renal cysts. As always, the TCG is set to give a uniform echo density throughout the picture.

SCANNING HINTS

Having gotten the patient positioned properly, we are ready to make the first transverse scan. "How will I recognize the kidney?" you may be wondering. Well, it is not difficult because the kidney has a really distinctive ultrasonic appearance. It has been compared to many things: a coffee bean, for example.

Figure 8–6. When the gain is properly adjusted the renal parenchyma should be light gray and the echoes from the central collecting system dark.

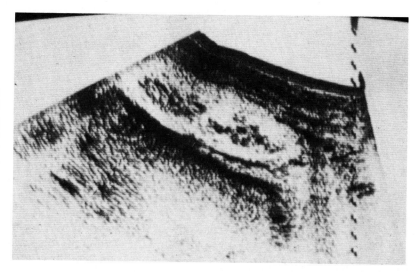

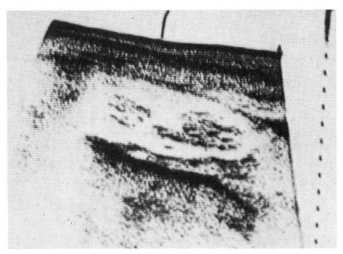

Figure 8–7. The gain must be set high enough to record echoes from the renal parenchyma. In this scan (the same kidney as in Figure 8–6) the gain is too low; there are no echoes from the kidney and a small lesion could be missed.

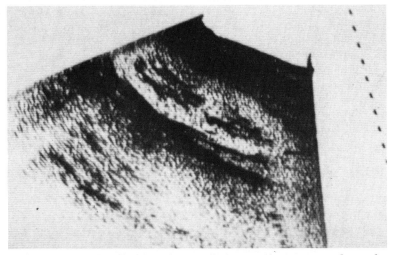

Figure 8–8. If the gain is set too high, artifacts will obscure the picture. This is the same kidney as in Figure 8–6 but the gain is too high.

Put into more scientific terms, the outer part of the kidney, including those portions which the anatomists call the cortex and the medulla (and which we call the parenchyma) is generally smooth, rather uniform in thickness, and produces very weak echoes. The central part of the kidney, where the collecting system and the larger blood vessels are found, contains many very strong echoes. These central echoes are usually bunched together and are not normally separated by any echo-free areas.

In the transverse section, the shape of the kidney is usually more or less round with the pelvic hilar structures oriented somewhat obliquely—the more medial portion being more anterior than the lateral. It is always the relatively echo-free parenchymal zone which seems to catch the eye as you scan; sometimes, in fact, the hilar structures do not appear without some effort (Fig. 8–9).

When making transverse scans, as a rule we begin medially toward the middle of the back and move the transducer laterally.

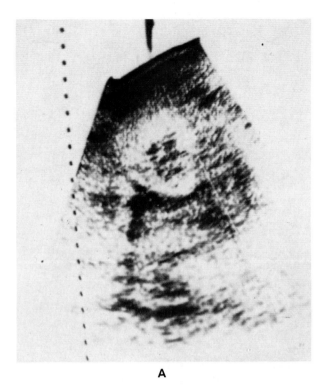

A

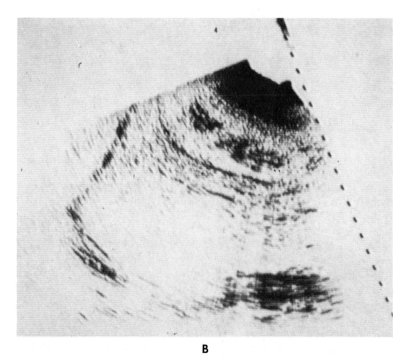

B

Figure 8–9. The kidney has a quite typical appearance. The parenchyma is relatively light gray; the central hilar structures (vessels and pelvis) are much darker gray.

A, Transverse section of normal left kidney.

B, Longitudinal section of normal left kidney.

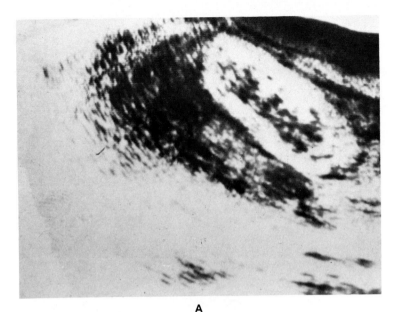

A

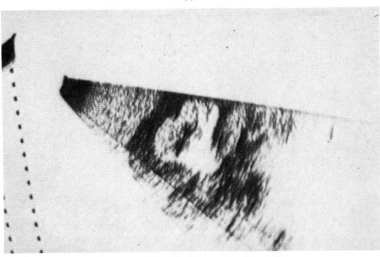

B

Figure 8–10. It is important to keep the transducer over an acoustic window when scanning the kidneys.

A, Sometimes the acoustic window is large, as in this case: the kidney can be easily outlined.

B, The upper pole of this kidney, containing a small cyst, could be visualized only on a sector scan between two ribs with the patient supine.

We usually sector-scan once the kidney is identified; that is, we angle the transducer from medial to lateral, keeping it in a spot over the midpoint of the kidney. As always, an effort is made to avoid scanning the kidney itself more than once on the same scan. Remember that scanning is harmless and it is cheap; do not hesitate to repeat a scan several times while experimenting with changes in gain, transducer motion, and so on, until you get a scan that is technically pleasing. You can then record the image on film.

Sometimes when doing transverse scans we will be examining one of the poles of the kidney and miss pelvic structures completely. In this case, the renal parenchyma is still apparent, and we are able to recognize the kidney as a round, relatively echo-free zone. Moving up or down the long axis of the kidney and making another scan will help confirm that we are indeed looking at the kidney. A reminder: sectoring is important when scanning the kidney, because the acoustic window is relatively limited, especially toward the upper pole. The

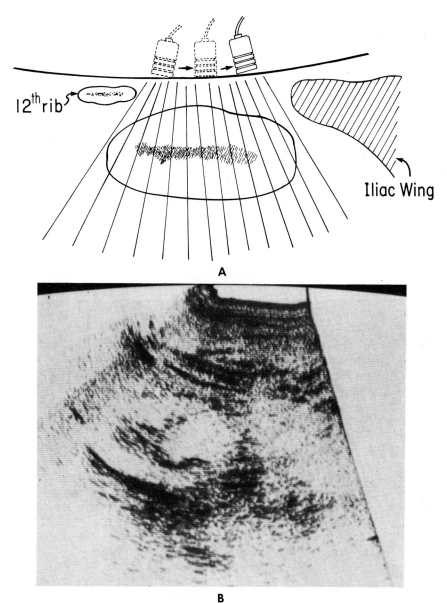

A

B

Figure 8–11. The poles of the kidney are often hidden beneath the twelfth rib or iliac crest. In these situations the sound beam must be sharply angled so that it does not pass through bone.

A, A diagrammatic representation of the acoustic window for the kidney.

B, A longitudinal renal scan made through a small window; the transducer has to be angled sharply up underneath the twelfth rib (notice the tumor in the lower pole).

problem is that one runs into the vertebral column medially and the lower ribs laterally. It is only through the window provided by the muscular paraspinal area that one can get a satisfactory look at the organ (Fig. 8–10).

Once we have obtained transverse scans, we move on to the longitudinal views. Ideally, we try to define both poles as well as the pelvic structures on each longitudinal scan. Here again the renal parenchyma is light gray, and the central structures are seen as a cluster of strong black echoes. We make a series of scans beginning medially and moving across the kidney in 1 centimeter steps, so that in the end there are usually three or four longitudinal scans. Because the upper pole is often hidden by the ribs, it is usually necessary to angle the sound beam rather sharply toward the head to see the upper pole clearly, as illustrated in Figure 8–11. If the upper pole cannot be demonstrated adequately by this maneuver, the transducer should be placed between the eleventh and twelfth ribs and a sector scan performed in that position. Remember, respiratory motion will obscure subtle lesions.

CLINICAL UTILITY

Almost invariably, renal lesions are first noted on an intravenous pyelogram (IVP). It is seldom that a renal ultrasound scan will be requested unless an IVP has been done first. Occasionally, however, a patient is known to be allergic to the contrast agent, and there are other patients whose renal function is so poor that the kidneys are not visible on the X-ray. In these instances it may be necessary to do renal ultrasound scans without the advantage of the X-ray study. Assuming that an IVP is available, however, it is always wise to consult the X-rays first to determine the position of the kidneys, where any lesions are located, and what specific information is sought. Once we have in mind what we are looking for, we are in good position to work out the problem.

What questions can be answered by ultrasound scanning? We have found that ultrasound is best at answering questions relating to a mass, especially if the mass is enlarging the renal outline in a particular area. In other words, it is much easier to evaluate a peripheral lesion than one which is located near the center of the kidney. Obviously, the larger a mass is, the easier it is to identify. We can differentiate between a cyst and a solid tumor (a polite word generally used to mean cancer, the commonest cause of tumor). Often, we can tell that a lump seen on the IVP is really a cyst and will not have to be evaluated by arteriogram. Renal cysts are totally echo-free — more so than the normal renal parenchyma. Usually cysts enlarge the outline of the kidney itself; and this, together with the diminished echo activity, makes them very easy to locate. On the other hand, renal tumors are more or less solid; this means, of course, that there will be echoes within a tumor or cancer, and they are frequently inhomogeneous. (Bear in mind that ultrasound shows primarily texture.) The cyst is really just a bag of water, while a tumor is more like an orange with inter-faces within it to produce echoes; the ultrasound images reflect this difference. Of course, there may be more than one lesion within the same kidney; thus it is important to recall the IVP findings, so as not to overlook a second or third lesion. Although it may be good for the ego to play games when scanning to see how well you can do with ultrasound alone, failure to make use of the radiographic information does not serve the patient's best interest in the long run.

One of the most frequent questions you will be asked is "How small a lesion can you find?" This type of question leads to claims and counterclaims as to what method is best for evaluating renal masses. There is no easy answer to this. If there is a cyst on the outer edge of the kidney, it can be seen with ultrasound, even if quite small — 1 centimeter, for example. On the other hand, a 1-centimeter cyst located adjacent to the renal pelvis will be impossible to distinguish from the normal renal collecting system or renal vein. In general, a tumor will be similar to the adjacent renal parenchyma. Any mass will be harder to find in a lumpy kidney. If there are multiple masses, it may be difficult to be certain which one you are looking at. So where does ultrasound stand in this "resolution" rat race? Right in the middle, we believe. Certainly ultrasound has better resolution than a renal isotope scan or a computed tomogram, but we feel that a well done intravenous pyelogram beats them all. In the presence of a normal IVP which is of satisfactory technical quality, we do not think ultrasound will uncover anything new. If the IVP is abnormal or equivocal, however, ultrasound is the next logical examination.

If a lesion is determined to be cystic, the next step is usually aspiration of the cyst. In simple terms, this means sticking a needle into it and sucking out some of the fluid it contains for study. This procedure demonstrates one of the fundamental rules of modern medicine: as soon as possible convert a noninvasive study into an invasive study; it is much more convincing and dramatic for all concerned. Aspiration of a cyst, of course, is not new; for a decade or so renal cyst aspiration under fluoroscopic guidance has been the standard method of definitive evaluation of these lesions. It has been determined that there is a slight chance—less then one in a hundred cases—that a cyst will harbor a cancer.

The reason for doing a cyst puncture, then, is to obtain some fluid for cytologic and chemical examination (qualitative fat and leucine dehyrogenase, or LDH, activity), and in some institutions further radiologic assessment of the interior of the cyst is performed after a small volume (5 to 10 ml) of water-soluble iodinated contrast agent (Hypaque or Renografin) and 20 to 40 cc of room air are injected.

Whenever possible, renal cyst puncture should be performed under ultrasonic guidance. Ultrasound has several advantages over fluoroscopy: no contrast is needed, no radiation is given to either patient or physician, and, most importantly, the depth of the cyst can be accurately determined by ultrasound. The procedure for ultrasonically guided aspiration will be described in detail in Chapter 13. Renal cyst puncture is an innocuous maneuver which patients tolerate very well; there is little pain, and there have been few complications. There may be a theoretic reason for avoiding a mass closely related to the renal pelvis for fear of entering either the collecting system or a major renal vessel. This has proved not to be a significant danger because a cutting needle is not used, and the diameter of the needle is quite small (21 to 23 gauge). We view this procedure as one for the physician to perform. It is really beyond the area of responsibility for the technologist, more from the standpoint of ethical and medico-legal aspects than anything else; but it is, nonetheless, outside the scope of technologists' practice.

Aspiration of solid renal masses for cytologic evaluation can also be done with ease and impunity. If cancer is confirmed by ultrasound examination, however, it is almost certain that surgical removal of the cancerous kidney will be performed. In many cases the surgeon will want to know about the blood supply and the possible involvement of renal vein, and he may want preoperative embolization performed. For these reasons, we feel that after conventional ultrasound scanning the next radiologic step in the assessment of a solid renal tumor is generally arteriography. We do not, however, hesitate to aspirate solid renal masses when a "tissue" diagnosis is sought in cases where nephrectomy will *not* be carried out.

One last word about conventional renal biopsy: ultrasound is a very convenient way for guiding the standard "cutting needle" when a renal biopsy is done. In this instance, the objective is to obtain a core of renal parenchyma to aid in the diagnosis of renal disease, not in the assessment of a renal mass. Ultrasound is especially useful when the renal function is so poor that the kidneys cannot be seen fluoroscopically. It is not difficult to locate the lower pole of the kidney and indicate where and how deep the needle should be introduced.

Hydronephrosis is another diagnosis which can be easily made by ultrasound. Here the renal parenchyma is generally normal, but the central hilar echoes are separated by echo-free spaces, and the dilated pelvis itself can be recognized as an echo-free zone medially. In these cases, ultrasound provides the most direct route to the proper diagnosis, because it can be performed with no preparation, is noninvasive, and does not require that the kidneys be functioning. The pelvis in such cases is really a cyst and is, therefore, easily recognized when dilated. In severe obstruction, excretion of intravenously administered contrast agent may be so limited that opacification of the collecting system will not be adequate for detailed evaluation. It is also possible to guide the placement of a catheter into the dilated renal pelvis so that contrast material can be injected directly for clearer assessment of the pelvis and the proximal ureter. Finally, sometimes an obstructed collecting system has to be drained for the sake of treating an infection. Using the same technique as outlined above, catheters for drainage can be placed quite easily under ultrasonic guidance.

The use of A-mode is frequently recommended as a means of differentiating betweeen solid and cystic masses in kidneys. It is a simple matter to switch from B- to A-mode with the sound beam passing through the area in question. The gain is then varied to see what pattern of echoes develops within the mass. We no longer use this technique because the advent of gray scale imaging has made it unnecessary to resort to A-mode. If the gain is set properly, there will usually be a clear difference between cystic and solid renal lesions on the B-scan itself.

Finally, ultrasound is an accurate method for measuring both renal size and volume. This is particularly important in following patients who have had a renal transplant, because it has been observed that an acute increase in the size of the grafted kidney is evidence of rejection crisis. The actual details of this calculation are somewhat more complex than is appropriate for this discussion. It is enough to say that the volume can be derived by a rather simple geometric calculation based on both longitudinal and transverse scans.

But enough about the kidney—go catch one to work on. Soon you will be thrilled to see lovely images looking at you from the television screen, as easy as one, two, three.

Chapter 9

EXAMINATION OF THE PELVIS

The pelvis is another area where ultra-sound has brought a rather dramatic advance in diagnostic capabilities, because there is really no other convenient means of getting a direct look at most of the structures there. This does not mean that there are no difficulties in the ultrasonic assessment of the pelvis; as always, however, there are some simple rules which help us. We are going to concern ourselves in this chapter with problems that have to do for the most part with conditions other than pregnancy. The examination of the gravid uterus will be covered in Chapter 10. In some instances early pregnancy will be dealt with here, but usually only because it is involved in the differential diagnosis of various pelvic conditions. Also, the male pelvis will get little attention. We are not being sexist; it is simply a fact that questions of pelvic disease are not common in the male.

SET UP, PREPARATION, AND TECHNIQUE

Without an acoustic window, there is almost no chance of your ever seeing into the pelvis with ultrasound; therefore, the filled urinary bladder is an absolute must. We have said this before, and you will hear it again; when undergoing examination of the pelvis, patients must not be studied unless the bladder is distended and this usually means uncomfortably full. If you put the patient on the table and find the bladder is empty, take a deep breath, explain the situation politely, and take her off the table. If it is not medically forbidden, hand the patient several glasses of water (or some other more attractive liquid if available) and try again in about 30 to 45 minutes. Of course,

there are some exceptions to this as to any arbitrarily stated rule, particularly if you are dealing with a huge pelvic mass such as an ovarian cyst; and perhaps it will be worth your while to make at least one midline longitudinal scan before going through your water routine. We are trying to emphasize, however, that generally speaking, you will need that acoustic window to get the information that you seek.

In some instances the patient may have an indwelling bladder catheter. It is then possible to distend the bladder by instilling sterile saline, not water, carefully under sterile conditions. Before trying this, be sure that you understand clearly what the patient's problem is; you would not want to fill up the bladder if there were reason to suspect that the integrity of the bladder wall was compromised. We urge you, therefore, to ask the patient's physician for permission to fill the bladder in this retrograde manner.

Before you start the study, there are a few other important items, all pertaining to history. In the pelvis, probably more than anyplace else in the body, we are dependent upon the history for guidance. We simply must have a clear idea of what the clinician is looking for if we are to be able to interpret the data we get. Not every question of history will be applicable to every patient; nevertheless, before starting you should determine such things as: Does the patient have a positive test for pregnancy? Is an intrauterine contraceptive device (IUD) known to be somewhere in the pelvis by previous x-ray? What has the referring physician found on physical examination? Has the patient undergone recent surgery? Are there any pelvic calcifications? Is the patient febrile or the white blood cell count elevated? Now, the way to get this information is to go through the chart or require pertinent data from the physician who sends the patient to you. You might also ask a few questions of the patient; it is surprising how well they often understand things. There is no easy way around the need for this background; without it you will be in trouble.

We do not deviate from standard abdominal technique when looking at the pelvis. Again, the 2.25 MHz, 19 mm diameter transducer with long internal focus is used. Often the 2:1 scale will be helpful, because the area covered by the scan is not great, and things usually fit well into that format. Because the anatomy is much easier to define on longitudinal sections than it is on transverse ones, we always begin longitudinally, moving the transducer in a modified sector scan so that the bladder can be used as a window as far cranially as possible (Fig. 9–1). We scan in the mid-line and to right and left, encompassing all of the pelvis as far laterally as the pelvic walls. The transverse scans usually are done with the transducer angled cephalad, for several reasons. The angulation helps "stretch" the window so that we can see farther up into the lower abdomen. Also, if you glance at Figure 9–1 again, you will see that the uterus is angled somewhat an-

teriorly. Tilting the plane of the transverse scan allows us to cut across the uterus more or less perpendicular to its long axis, and this produces images which are somewhat easier to understand. Again, modified sectoring is usually the order of the day, because by this means we can use our window to look at the lateral walls of the pelvis (Fig. 9–2). We make as many transverse cuts as we feel are necessary to investigate the entire pelvis; usually two or three are the minimum.

We should mention one problem which can arise in either sex and can mislead you; namely, the presence of feces in the rectum and sigmoid colon. If there is little gas present, bowel content can easily simulate a mass by appearing as a relatively echo-free area. Usually the location of the "mass" is the tip-off that you are being fooled by feces in colon; because when this artifact does occur, it is almost always found posteriorly or to the left. If you encounter such a finding and are smart enough to tumble to the possibility of its being an artifact, you can then test your thesis by emptying the colon. We will leave the technique of this to your imagination; remember, however, that if there is a question of intestinal obstruction or inflammation, it may not be wise to give the

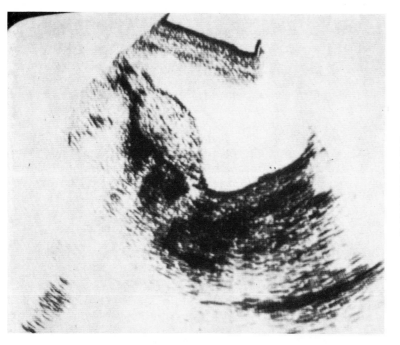

Figure 9–1. Pelvic anatomy is easiest to recognize in longitudinal scans. This midline (L,0) scan shows the normal relationship of the bladder and uterus. The patient's bladder must be full to provide an acoustic window into the pelvis.

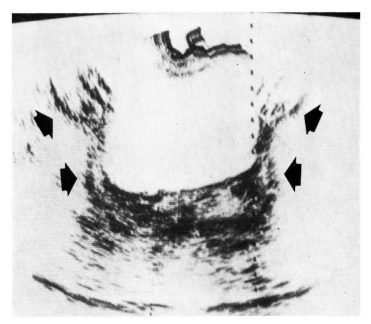

Figure 9-2. A full bladder permits the entire pelvis to be visualized. This transverse section shows not only the neck of the uterus and left adnexal mass but also the side walls of the pelvis (*arrows*).

patient an enema. Under these circumstances, then, we suggest you check with the referring physician. If you do not want to get into the business of giving enemas, etc., in the ultrasound lab (and we avoid this ourselves) you can always ask the clinician involved to arrange to have the patient's colon cleaned out and repeat the study at another time.

SPECIFIC EXAMINATIONS

The Uterus

In more ways than one the uterus is the central organ of the pelvis and figures in almost all clinical situations arising in this area in women. The normal uterus is easy to recognize because on the longitu-

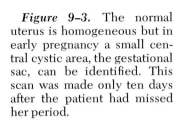

Figure 9-3. The normal uterus is homogeneous but in early pregnancy a small central cystic area, the gestational sac, can be identified. This scan was made only ten days after the patient had missed her period.

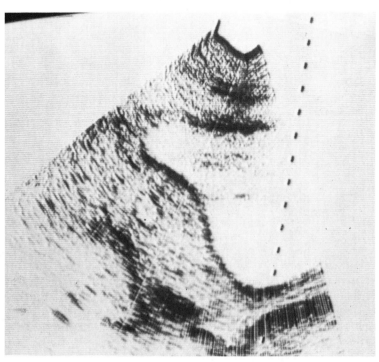

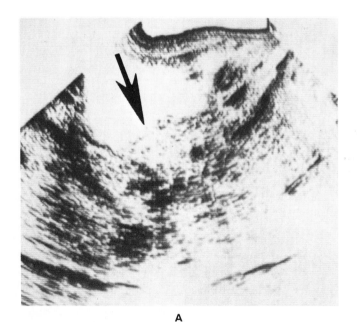

A

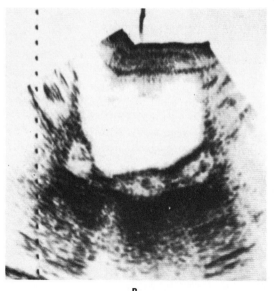

B

Figure 9–4. The uterus is larger in the fundus than in the neck.

A, A transverse section through the uterine fundus (*arrow*). (The amorphous echoes to the right—*the patient's right*—of the uterus are from the patient's adnexa.)

B, A transverse section through the uterine neck; notice the ovaries on either side of the uterus. The dark echo in the center of the uterus is from a portion of an IUD.

dinal scan it usually lies obliquely behind the urinary bladder and is flecked with relatively weak internal echoes (Fig. 9–1). During pregnancy the uterus enlarges very quickly, and from about six weeks after the start of the last normal menstrual period, an echo-free zone (the gestational sac) can be seen within it (Fig. 9–3). If the patient is known to be pregnant, then identification of the gestational sac in the uterus is an important goal of the ultrasonographer, particularly if there is a question of an ectopic pregnancy (that is, a pregnancy outside of the uterus). In the nonpregnant uterus the shape and size of the organ is important.

We do not like to set forth numbers for measurement and will not do so here; it is enough to say that the size of the normal uterus will become familiar to you as you gain experience, and you will also come to appreciate that it is usually smooth and elliptical in contour. Transversely, the uterus is more or less round in cross-section, narrower down toward the cervix than in the fundus (Fig. 9–4).

These days there is a fair amount of attention given to birth control; so almost anywhere you work, if you have any obstetrical or gynecological business at all, you will be asked soon to locate an IUD which

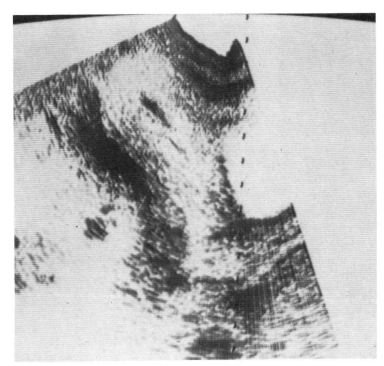

Figure 9–5. When an IUD is correctly positioned within the uterine cavity, it produces loud echoes which are not normally present (cf. Figure 9–1). This uterus is normal in size but appears large because the bladder is nearly empty.

the patient or her doctor cannot find. This chore can be a bit tricky. If there is no question of pregnancy, we like to have an X-ray film of the pelvis done first. This will show if the IUD is present or not. If it is present on the film, or if the patient is pregnant, a pelvic ultrasound scan is done to see if the IUD can be located (Fig. 9–5). Generally speaking, these little items produce linear, rather strong, nonanatomic echoes which allow the IUD to be identified. Looking blindly for them can be troublesome, however, so if the clinical circumstances allow you to get an X-ray, do so. Your objective is to decide where the IUD is: intra- or extrauterine, or perhaps a bit of both.

The Ovaries and Adnexae

The normal ovaries and the structures lateral to the uterus are difficult to appreciate when scanning longitudinally, so we will concentrate our attention on the transverse scan. Sometimes the normal ovaries can be seen lateral to the uterus as relatively echo-free circles within the rather dense echo-producing structures of the ad-

nexae (Fig. 9–6). If you see normal ovaries, consider yourself lucky. Almost always when an ovary is seen well, it is because it is enlarged by tumor, cysts, or infection. By the same token, if the adnexae do not have the monotonous inhomogeneity which produces dense echoes, that is, if a relatively echo-free area is visualized lateral to the uterus, it is almost certain that some pathologic condition is present. Infection, bleeding, or tumor all tend to decrease echo production so that they will be seen as relatively echo-free areas. While it is not so difficult to appreciate that an abnormality is present, it is something else again to decide what the pathologic process is without help from the physical examination or laboratory data (Fig. 9–7). If things go right and you have a satisfactory look, the lateral pelvic walls will be visible, an important feature of the examination if we are trying to exclude postoperative infection or define extension of malignancy.

Putting all of this together, then, in our examination of the female pelvis, what can we offer the referring physician? Well, we can easily find, or, more important, perhaps, verify the presence of a pelvic mass. We can tell if this mass is cystic or solid.

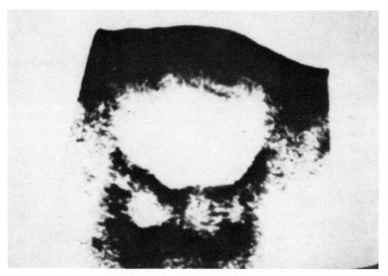

Figure 9–6. It is not always possible to visualize normal-sized ovaries. This transverse section through the ovaries demonstrates the uterus, a normal left ovary, and a small corpus luteum cyst in the right ovary.

We can show how large the mass is and what structures it involves or invades. Together with the clinical and laboratory data, this usually permits a fairly specific diagnosis.

Urinary Bladder

We have spoken of the importance of the urinary bladder as a transmitter of sound, our "window on the pelvis" as it were; but we should bear in mind that ultrasound can be helpful in evaluating the bladder itself. With a little geometry and the help of the computer, it is possible to calculate the volume of the bladder—a pleasant exercise in mathematics for some, but not particularly useful from the clinical standpoint. The bladder wall is easily defined so that abnormalities can be seen, usually as irregularity or thickening; and it is possible to document the presence of bladder stones or other foreign bodies. What is more, you may discover, once you have begun scanning, that you are the first to recognize that the patient you are examining has a large, distended bladder, not previously noted. This may seem to be an exotic way to diagnose urinary retention; but information is information, and you will want to pass it on to the patient's physician.

Prostate

Finally there is the matter of the prostate. We have had little experience visualizing this gland ultrasonically, and we have little to say beyond the fact that it is not widely done in clinical practice as yet. Japanese ultrasonographers have built special transducers for examining the prostate transrectally, and they show the relationship of the prostate to rectum and pelvic walls quite clearly. Most of us do not have this specialized apparatus and may never have it, so we have tried to see the prostate both longitudinally and transversely (with the sound beam angled toward the feet). This technique produces a remarkably good image of the gland and may allow you to estimate its size and the possible extension of tumor, if present, toward the pelvic wall (Fig. 9–8). Some ultrasonographers recommend placing the transducer on the perineum and scanning upward; we have no experience with this method. The prostate is inhomogeneous and, therefore, is not echo-free; so it is not possible to distinguish between adenomatous and malignant disease. If an abscess were present, however, it would be recognizable by conventional scanning as an area of relatively diminished echo production.

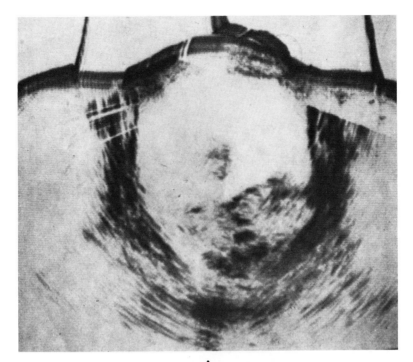

A

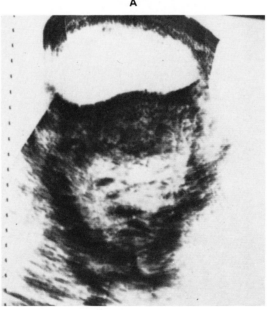

B

Figure 9–7. It is not possible to make a specific pathologic diagnosis based on the ultrasound appearance alone.

A, A transverse scan showing a complex mass in the cul-de-sac, underneath the bladder—this was a carcinoma of the ovary. (Ignore the artifact in the bladder.)

B, A transverse scan in a patient with pelvic inflammatory disease and cul-de-sac inflammation and abscesses.

Although the appearance of these two scans is nearly identical, the diagnosis was very different: ectopic pregnancy and some types of benign ovarian tumors can also look just like this. Fortunately, the combination of clinical data, physical examination, and ultrasound often permits a specific diagnosis to be made.

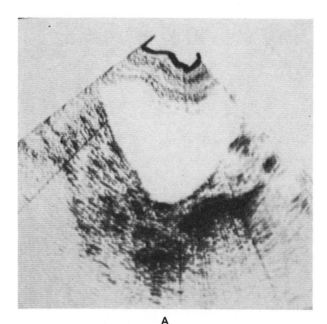

A

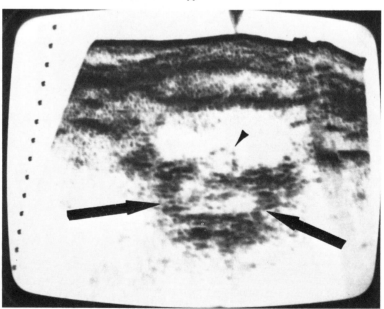

B

Figure 9–8. The prostate can often be visualized if the bladder is used as an acoustic window. A, Longitudinal scan of a normal prostate.

B, A cross-section scan of a prostate tumor—a rhabdomyosarcoma (*large arrows*). Notice the echoes from tumor extension into the bladder (*arrowhead*). The tumor does not involve the walls of the pelvis.

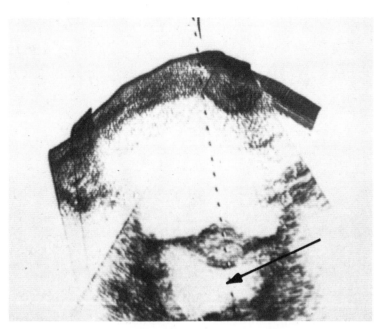

Figure 9–9. Ascitic fluid collects in the pelvis where it is readily identified. This transverse scan of a patient with ascites shows the bladder and the pool of ascitic fluid posteriorly, the two separated by the uterus and broad ligaments. Arrow points to the ascites in the cul-de-sac.

One further word about the pelvis in general; as every radiologist knows, ascitic fluid in the belly collects in the true pelvis when the patient is supine. The same phenomenon which creates the relatively uniform density in the pelvis of an abdomen with ascites on the X-ray will produce an easily appreciated echo-free zone behind the urinary bladder when scanned by ultrasound (Fig. 9–9). A small volume of intraperitoneal fluid may be very hard to pick up by physical examination, but it will not pose much of a problem for ultrasound—provided, of course, as always, the filled urinary bladder is there to allow us to see into the pelvis.

Chapter 10

EXAMINATION IN PREGNANCY

How many times have you heard it said that obstetrics must be such a *nice* specialty because one is always working with happy, healthy, young patients; and you, hardened cynic that you are, felt like throwing up at once? Well, get out the wastebasket or head for the john, because here comes the same sentiment: obstetrics *is* fun for the ultrasonographer, not only because these patients are usually pleasant to deal with, but also because there is no more ideal target for ultrasound than the pregnant uterus. Because things can be seen so well with little or no effort and few artifacts arise to louse up the study, it is a very satisfying experience to examine a pregnancy. In obstetrics ultrasound has almost completely supplanted older means of visualizing the uterus (radionuclide placentography, and gestational dating by radiographic epiphyseal assessment, for example); and, in fact, ultrasound provides information not easily obtained by any other noninvasive procedure.

SET UP AND PREPARATION

The study of the uterus has to be tailored somewhat to the stage of gestation; however, there are some fundamental principles which apply; and as we go along, we will indicate where deviation has to be made. Let us remind you to insist that the patient come to the ultrasound lab with a full urinary bladder. (By now, this is a very tired tune, we know; but we play it again to emphasize the value of the bladder as an acoustic window in obstetrics as in all cases where it is necessary to look into the pelvis.) Having the urinary bladder distended is of paramount importance in early pregnancy (say, up to 20 weeks' gestation);

because until the uterus is greatly enlarged, small bowel will overlie it in the pelvis, and gas will frequently obscure things. Even later in pregnancy a full bladder can help to visualize the lower uterine segment, especially in instances where locating the placenta is difficult. So, we prepare obstetrical patients by having them go for about four hours without urinating. Other than this, no preparation is needed; the patient does not have to fast.

This is certainly one time when our patients are glad that we have gone to some trouble to provide them with a comfortable examining table, because women are usually more than just a bit uncomfortable toward the end of pregnancy. Often, after lying supine for a few minutes, the patient will become restless and sweaty and will soon complain of feeling faint and nauseated. This happens because blood flow to the heart is blocked by the pressure of the uterus on the inferior vena cava (IVC). To cure it, all we need to do is turn the patient slightly (10° to 15°) to either side. We use a foam rubber wedge such as the one used to position patients for oblique views of the lumbar spine; when placed under one hip to get the patient off her back, this will usually relieve the symptoms quickly. We do not turn the patient unless trouble develops because it is more convenient not to have to contend with the angulations of the scanning head that this positioning requires.

For obstetrical scanning we use almost exclusively the 2.25 MHz, 19 mm diameter transducer with long internal focus which is standard for all abdominal examinations. The gain and TGC settings are also similar to those for the abdomen. (Ideally they are adjusted so that the echo strengths are more or less the same throughout the depth of the uterus and the fluid-bearing areas are clean and echo-free.) Once the proper setting is determined, little variation will be needed for the rest of the examination. In the main, we use the 3:1 scale; but here again, a larger scale (2:1) is used for study of earlier gestations (up to about 20 weeks) and recording for measurement of the fetal head.

SAFETY

In Chapter 1, we discussed the safety of ultrasound, but we want to remind everyone that, as far as can be determined, no harm is done to operator, mother, or child in scanning the pregnant uterus with B-mode ultrasound. What is more, there is no apparent limit to the number or frequency of studies that may be done during the same pregnancy, nor to the number of scans per examination. Remember that the commercial B-mode scanner uses pulsed sound, so that the machine is "listening" most of the time. Moreover, human tissue seems to have no memory for exposure to ultrasound of diagnostic frequency. In this respect, ultrasound affects tissue in a very different way from ionizing radiation. With X-ray exposure the tissue effect is never completely "forgotten." Finally, recall that ultrasound scanning in pregnancy is not a new technique; it has been used in countless thousands of pregnancies since being introduced into clinical practice in the late 1950's. Examination of the children of many of these pregnancies has failed to uncover any evidence of injury that might be related to the ultrasound, and the potential period of observation here has been nearly 20 years.

TECHNIQUE AND LANDMARKS

We have found it best to begin scanning longitudinally in the midline, no matter what the stage of gestation. Usually three scans longitudinally are the minimum needed to visualize the entire pelvis, and this will be sufficient only for the earliest pregnancies. Beyond 20 weeks' gestation it may be necessary to get as many as five or more longitudinal scans. The coordinate system set up for abdominal scanning is used here as well; that is, longitudinal

scans are tagged $L \pm X$ indicating displacement to right (+) or left (−) of midline $(L,0)$ and $C \pm X$ relating transverse planes to the iliac crest, above the crest being designated "+", below "−". The scanning motion used is a combination of sectoring and simple sweeping; sectoring may be needed particularly at the fundus where intestinal gas may be encountered and just above the symphysis to enable us to see behind and below that bone. There are a number of landmarks we must identify to be certain that the examination is satisfactory, and they will vary considerably with the age of gestation. Let us begin by taking a look at pregnancy at about eight weeks' gestation, that is, eight weeks since the onset of the last normal menstrual period (LNMP).

Maybe we should stop for a moment to say a word or two about the term "gestational age." Normally, women ovulate about two weeks after the start of the menstrual period. It is only after ovulation that conception can occur, and then gestation begins. This means that the fetus is usually about two weeks "younger" than the gestational age. To put some numbers on this, if a woman's periods come every 28 days, at the time of her first missed period, the gestation is four weeks of age. Assuming that she ovulated two weeks after the onset of her last period, the fetus is two weeks of age. Because by convention all the dates are figured from the LNMP, we use this gestational age when describing pregnancies; it is convenient and easy to calculate.

In the L,0 plane the cervix and the body of the uterus are seen (Fig. 10–1). The walls of the posterior vagina are sometimes seen as well. The body of the uterus contains a central echo-free zone, which is known as the gestational sac. This is surrounded by the rather thick, lightly flecked walls of the uterus. Lying anterior to the uterus is the echo-free urine-filled bladder.

(*Review question department:* What are the linear collections of dense echoes which are seen just beneath the anterior wall of the bladder? Remember from Chapter 5, they are reverberations; and they are very difficult to get rid of. Keep them in mind, because they are going to show up again soon.)

Recognizing the gestational sac is the *sine qua non* of the ultrasonic diagnosis of early pregnancy. It is possible to make this diagnosis with ultrasound by about six weeks after the LNMP. As weeks go by, linear echoes which actually arise from the fetus are seen; they are so small and nondescript that we cannot tell more than that they are present (Fig. 10–2). By about 13 weeks' gestation, however, the fetus has grown large enough so that the head is recognizable (Fig. 10–3). It is no trick to identify the head because of its shape and the straight line in the middle of it, probably produced by the falx cerebri (although there is some debate about this among ultrasonographers). During this period of development a collection of many echoes has appeared along one side of the gestational sac. This is the placenta. As time goes on and the uterus grows, the walls of the uterus will thin out and the placenta will become even more obvious.

Scanning on either side of midline defines the entire uterus for us; we lose the cervix but can see more of the uterine contents. Much has been made of the shape and the integrity of the wall of the gestational sac in the assessment of early pregnancy. Although such discussion is beyond the scope of this text, it is important to point out that one goal of the study is to determine whether or not any gestational sac seen is actually intrauterine. This usually proves to be easy and is done by carefully noting if the sac is surrounded by the wall of the uterus. An ectopic pregnancy, one which develops outside of the uterus, is always life-threatening to the mother because of the likelihood that it will burst and cause serious intraperitoneal bleeding. Moreover, if an ectopic pregnancy does go to term, there is obviously no way for the baby to be born without operative intervention.

We stick to our routine of beginning with longitudinal scans when looking at more advanced pregnancies as well. Here the landmarks are more readily seen, and the first order of business is deciding where the fetal head is located. The presentation of the fetus is an important piece of information to include in the report. This means doing a series of longitudinal scans parallel to the long axis; usually at least three, and maybe five, will be needed. Once these scans have been made and have been set out in sequence, you can piece together the fetal parts so that you will know how many fetuses are present, what their position is (that is, head up, down, or transverse), and where the fetal small parts (limbs) are.

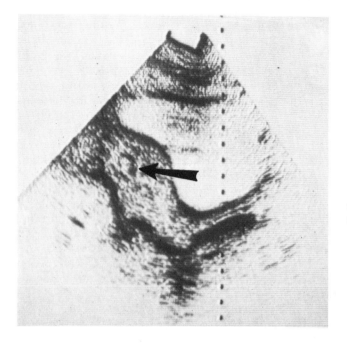

Figure 10–1. The earliest ultrasonic manifestation of pregnancy is the presence of a gestational sac within the uterine cavity *(arrow)*: the tiny sac in this uterus represented a five-week gestation. This midline (L,0) scan also shows the cervix and vagina.

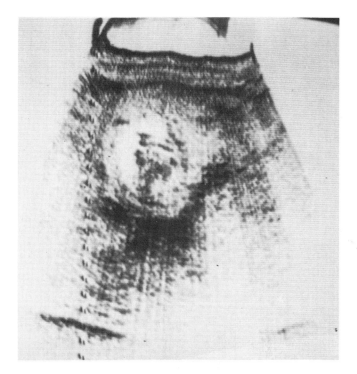

Figure 10-2. Between 10 and 13 weeks' gestational age the gestational sac evolves into the amniotic cavity, in which several internal echoes from the developing fetus are evident. There are no recognizable features at this stage, however. This is a transverse scan of an 11-week pregnancy.

At the same time you are putting the baby together in your mind's eye, you should locate the placenta (Fig. 10-4). If the placenta lies anteriorly, it will be easy to see. The fine speckling of its echo pattern and the well-defined line of the chorionic plate are unmistakable. If the placenta is posterior, however, it may be hidden partly or completely by the fetus (Fig. 10-5). Sometimes it cannot be clearly

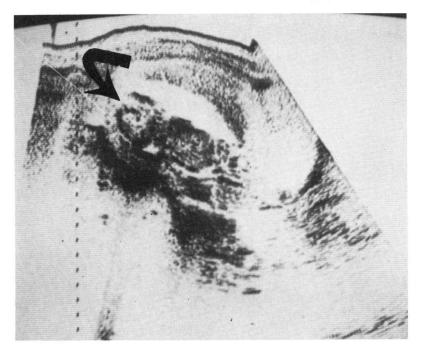

Figure 10-3. The fetal head and placenta are recognizable by 13 weeks' gestational age. This midline (L,0) scan shows the small fetal head (*curved arrow*) and the placenta on the anterior uterine wall.

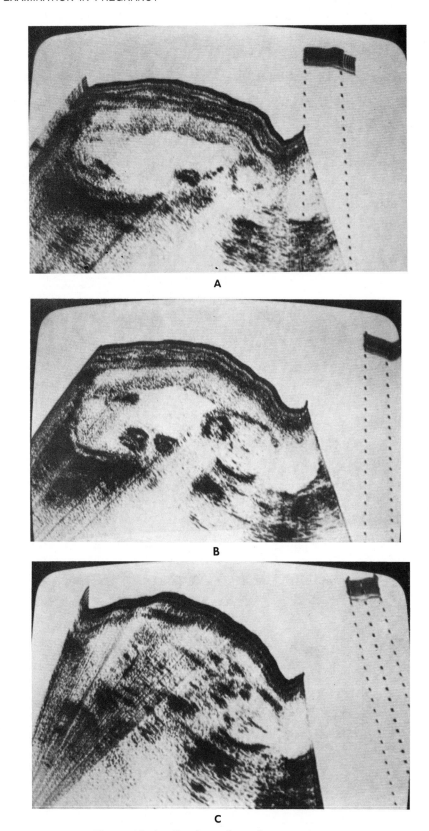

A

B

C

Figure 10–4. See legend on the opposite page.

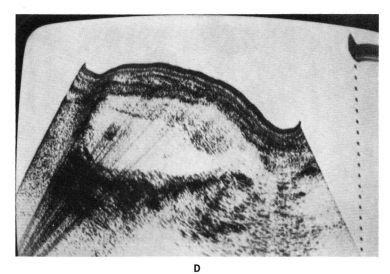

D

Figure 10–4. A mental image of the uterine contents can be constructed from a series of longitudinal scans. *A* to *D* are a series of scans made at L+4, L+2, L,0 and L–4 respectively. The fetus is in cephalic presentation with the head against the bladder; the fetal torso is in the midline and the arms and legs are directed to the right side. The placenta is clearly seen on the anterior uterine wall, slightly more prominent on the left side.

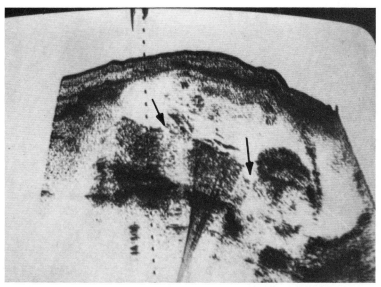

Figure 10–5. A posterior placenta can be difficult to identify completely because the overlying fetus interrupts the sound beam. In this L,0 scan we can easily identify some portions of the posterior placenta but fetal shadowing obscures the midportion and the distal margin (*arrows*).

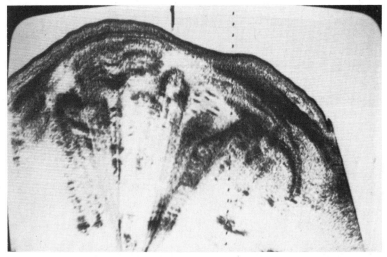

Figure 10-6. In the third trimester the fetus may completely obscure the posterior placenta, as shown in this L,0 scan. We can infer that there is a posterior placenta because the fetus is positioned anteriorly, adjacent to the uterine wall.

seen, but its position is known because the fetus is displaced away from the posterior uterine wall, and we can infer that the placenta must be causing this displacement (Fig. 10–6). We must define the lowest extent of the placenta in the midline longitudinal view to exclude the possibility of placenta previa. If the cervix can be seen well and we can show that the placenta ends well above it, this diagnosis is excluded (Fig. 10–7). Sometimes, of course, it is not possible to define the lower placental margin because it is obscured by the baby. Often we can show that the fetal head is so intimately applied to the cervix that there should be no room for the placenta, and placenta previa is excluded indirectly (Fig. 10–8).

In locating the placenta we again meet our old nemesis, the reverberation artifact, which sometimes simulates an anterior placenta (Fig. 10–9). Close observation gives us several clues as to the true nature of this phenomenon and helps us differentiate it from the placenta. First, we look for the placenta somewhere else. Then we note that there is no well-defined chorionic plate in the artifact, whereas the placenta is clearly limited by its plate. Finally, the reverberations parallel the anterior abdominal wall and may appear to be striped. The true placenta will often taper toward one end, and its thickness will not necessarily follow the contour of the belly wall.

We fill in with transverse sections some of the gaps in what we have already seen; probably three scans at a minimum. In early pregnancy, the lowest plane includes the cervix along with our friend the urinary bladder anteriorly (Fig. 10–10). Moving cranially, we encounter the body of the uterus and the gestational sac again (Fig. 10–11). In later pregnancy we choose scans which will pass through the fetal head and the fetal trunk at several levels (Fig. 10–12). Having made these scans, they too should be set out in sequence so that we can assemble in our mind a picture of how the fetus lies in the uterus and what the relationship of the placenta is to the fetus and the cervix (Fig. 10–13). *(Extra credit department:* It might be smart to draw out an actual picture as we have done after you have finished scanning. You will not find this useful in everyday practice, of course; but it is a good way to train yourself to synthesize your findings when you are first learning to scan.)

Text continued on page 167.

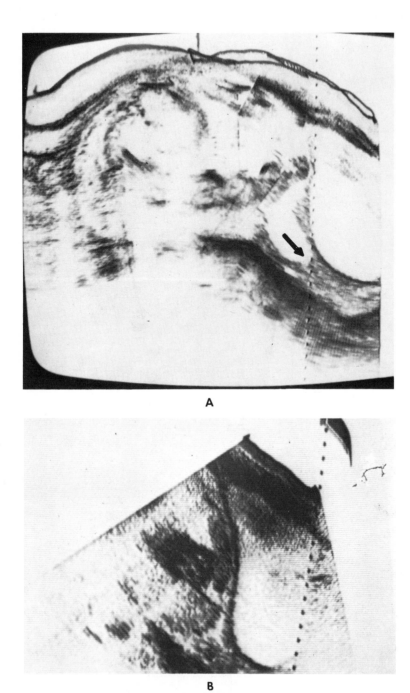

A

B

Figure 10-7. Placenta previa is defined by the relationship between the cervix and the edge of the placenta.

A, An L,0 scan: the placenta is on the posterior wall and extends into the fundus; there is only amniotic fluid adjacent to the internal cervical os (*arrow*).

B, An L,0 scan in a patient with placenta previa: the placenta is on the posterior wall but its edge extends across the cervical os.

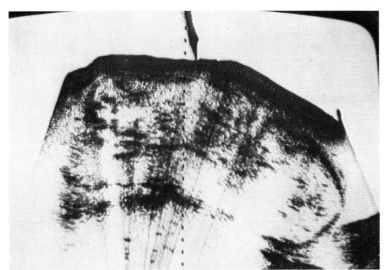

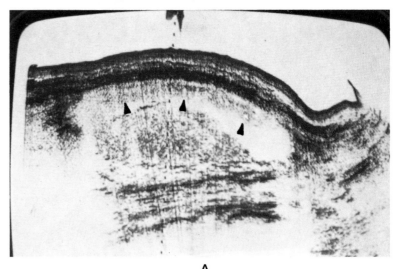

A

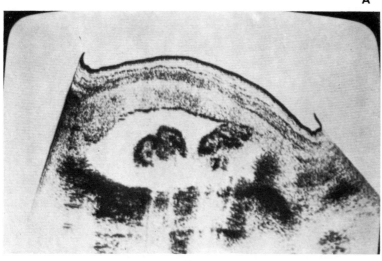

B

Figure 10–8. If the fetal head is against the cervical os, placenta previa can be excluded even if the placenta cannot be seen. In this L,0 scan the posterior placenta is not well visualized but the position of the fetal head makes us confident there is no placenta previa.

Figure 10–9. Reverberation artifacts may mimic an anterior placenta.

A, An L–3 scan with reverberation artifact *(arrowheads)* which could be mistaken for an anterior placenta: the actual placenta can be seen on the posterior wall.

B, An L–2 scan showing a true anterior placenta: the loud echo from the chorionic plate, which limits the placenta internally, helps differentiate the real placenta from artifacts.

162

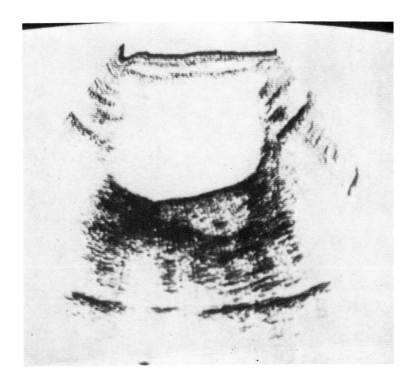

Figure 10–10. Low transverse sections show only the neck of the uterus or cervix and no evidence of a pregnancy higher in the uterus. This is a C–7, –20° scan.

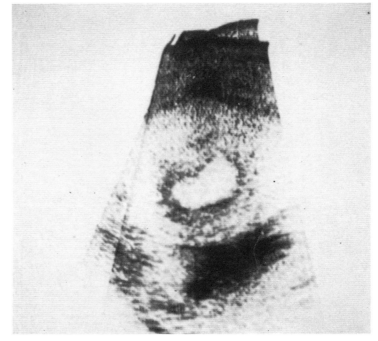

Figure 10–11. Transverse scans through the uterine fundus will demonstrate an intrauterine pregnancy. This 8-week gestational sac was scanned at C–2.

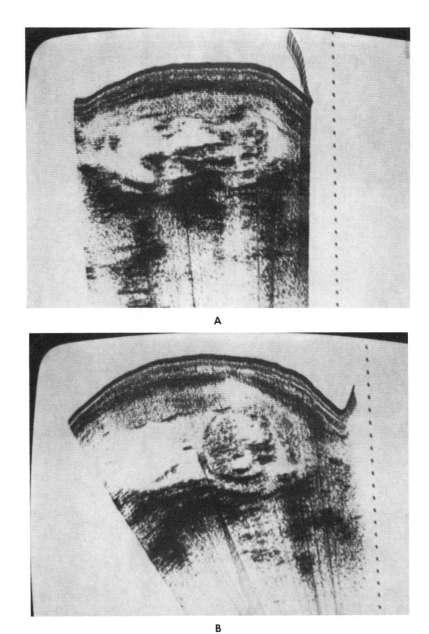

A

B

Figure 10–12. The arrangement of the uterine contents can be deduced from a series of transverse scans. *A* to *D* are a series of images obtained at C+6, C+2, C−2, and C−6 respectively. The presentation is cephalic, the back to the left and the placenta anterior.

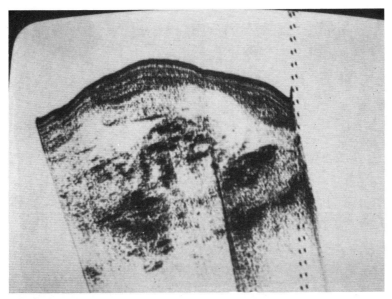

C

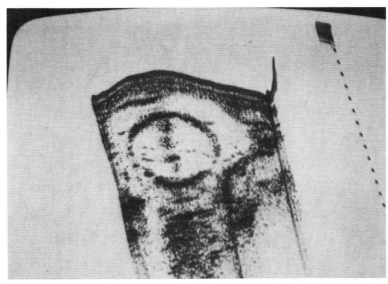

D

Figure 10–12 Continued.

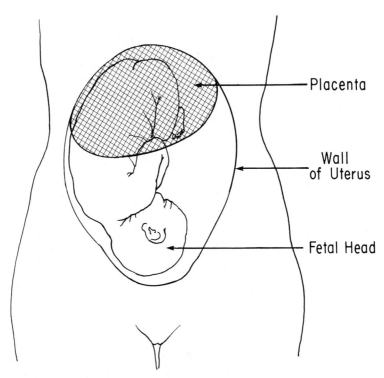

Figure 10–13. The ultrasonographer should construct a mental image of the arrangement of the uterine contents for each patient.

GESTATIONAL DATING

We have chosen to set apart several aspects of the obstetrical examination which are particularly important, and the first of these relates to the question of the determination of the age of pregnancy. Simply stated the question is: "When am I going to have my baby, Doctor?" Until you have become involved in the business of obstetrical care, you probably will have no idea how often patients are unsure of the date of conception. (Those of you who have children will probably not be surprised by this at all.) Nonetheless, now that we have a diagnostic technique which can give a rather precise estimate of gestational age, it is clear that the time of conception is often not recognized accurately by changes in menstrual periods. This does not mean that women are not observant of their bodily functions; more likely their periods or times of ovulation are variable, or they do not perceive subtle variation in their menstrual flow so that the onset of pregnancy is not appreciated. Also, there appears to be a group of women in whom physical examination is misleading, so that the examining physician is not able to judge reliably how far along a particular pregnancy has progressed. Finally, there are women who have underlying diseases which predispose them to obstetrical troubles (diabetes, hypertension, heart disease, blood factor sensitivity, to name a few). In these cases, failure of normal fetal growth may signal impending fetal death, and it is important to evaluate the fetus periodically to see that it is developing as expected. In all of the instances cited above, estimation of fetal age by ultrasound will provide the most accurate information available to the clinician.

Before the fetal head and parts are discernible, we estimate age by measuring the greatest diameter of the gestational sac. This means, of course, that the sac has to be well-defined and the centimeter markers flashed on the screen so that a frame of reference is available on the photograph. It is then a simple matter to take a small set of calipers (or the edge of a 3 × 5 inch card) and measure the diameter. (See the Bibliography for reference to a graph presenting the relationship of diameter of gestational sac and age.)

As the gestation progresses, there is some information that measurement of the crown-rump length is useful in making a more accurate estimate of fetal age. We have no experience with this, as we have not found it necessary to go beyond the sac for early dating. In fact, with a little experience you will find that you will be able to "eyeball" the gestational sac and arrive at a reasonable estimation of gestational age without referring to any table or graph. It is only sensible, however, to play it by the rules until you have gotten a good idea of how the uterus changes through the first trimester of pregnancy.

Almost always by 13 to 14 weeks of gestation, the fetal head can be seen. At this point it is possible to switch to using the biparietal diameter (BPD) of the fetal head to evaluate maturity. This procedure takes a little finesse because it relies on one's ability to display the fetal head as though viewed from above or from front or rear; and positioning has to be precise. Fortunately for us, the midplane of the skull is a nice reflector of sound, so that almost always we can produce a well-defined linear echo in the midline of the baby's head. The scanner is then angulated and moved, largely by trial and error, until this linear echo falls midway between the slightly curved lateral walls of the skull. Generally speaking, we do this manipulation while using gray scale. Once we have satisfied ourselves that we are scanning in a plane perpendicular to the sagittal or coronal planes of the fetal skull, we switch to bistable display. The gain is turned down until only the walls of the skull can be recorded and several scans are made. To be certain that we get a picture of the greatest BPD we move the scanning head in both directions while maintaining the same plane. Again, recording the scan on the largest possible scale (usually 2:1, but sometimes 1:1) and including the centimeter marker are important. This is an instance when the ultrasonographer has to use a bit of imagination to select the plane for scanning which will display the BPD most accurately. It always takes some fiddling with angulation, and it takes patience.

Having recorded the BPD in one plane, we turn the scanning head 90° (for example, from longitudinal to transverse) and go

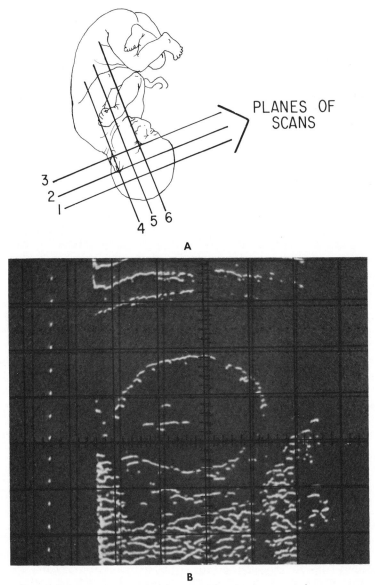

PLANES OF
SCANS

3
2
I
4 5 6

A

B

Figure 10–14. The biparietal diameter (BPD) should be measured in at least two different orientations. The shape of the skull will vary depending on whether a frontal or coronal section is obtained, but the BPD should be the same.

A, A diagrammatic representation of scanning planes for BPD measurements.

B, A coronal section: the skull is elliptical.

Legend continued on the opposite page

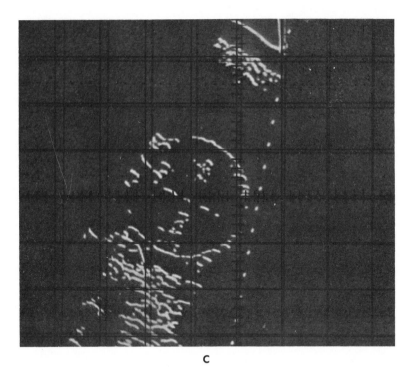

C

Figure 10–14 Continued. *C*, A frontal section of the same head as in *B*. The skull is round but the BPD measurement is the same as in *B*.

through the process in this plane (Fig. 10–14). The BPD measured in both positions should be the same; if not, the measurement has to be suspect. From our experience we believe that estimating fetal age is most reliable when done between the sixteenth and thirty-second weeks of gestation. There are several reasons for this. Probably the most important has to do with the fact that during this period the volume of amniotic fluid is great enough to provide a good acoustic window and the fetal head is usually positioned in such a way as to allow us to see it all. Before 16 weeks the fetal head is so small that it is difficult to make a picture of it; and after 32 weeks it is often so far down in the pelvis that it cannot be seen well. The fetal head grows more slowly after 30 weeks, and the difference in BPD as a function of fetal age decreases. Finally, a deeply engaged head has become molded and elliptical so that it is difficult to know where to make the measurements.

We do not use A-mode for fetal head measurement.

The availability of bi-stable facilitates recording a nice clean outline of the fetal skull; if you do not have this capability on your instrument, however, adjust the gain until the thinnest line possible is recorded.

We record a minimum of four BPD's (two in both planes). Often more are made and all are measured. We are more inclined to believe one scan which shows the midline echo symmetrically placed in a nice elliptical skull than several asymmetrical scans. Performing a good measurement of the fetal BPD calls for a fair measure of artistry and perseverance on the part of the ultrasonographer; do not despair if you encounter a bit of difficulty at first; here is certainly one instance when patience will help you greatly.

"What do I do with the BPD once I have measured it?" you ask. Very good. Well, obviously you will need a table giving gestational age as a function of BPD. (See Bibliography for some references in which tables are offered.) The validity of the relationship between the two has been well established by multiple studies. It has been noted that the relationship between BPD and gestational age does not vary significantly among different centers in the United States, Great Britain, and Europe; so that you will find it safe to borrow a table from someone else. Your estimate of gestational age should fall within a week on either side of the age determined by the date of the last LNMP. (Here is our own Catch-22: there is no foolproof way of knowing, of course, that the date given you by the patient was in fact her LNMP.) You can check your accuracy by keeping track of your patients; if your dating is correct, noninduced delivery should occur within one week of the estimated date of confinement you predict. (Remember, the normal gestation lasts 40 weeks from the onset of the LNMP.) If you are going to have a big obstetrical practice, it might be helpful to compare published tables against your own experience, so that you have a table which fits your particular patient population.

MULTIPLE GESTATION

The discovery of twins may strike terror in the hearts of the parents, but it proves to be great fun for the ultrasonographer. Unfortunately, however, any number of babies above two is likely to cause trouble in diagnosis, simply because there are so many fetal parts and it is difficult to sort them out. The trick is to visualize and identify accurately fetal heads and trunks; and while this may seem easy, wait until you have tried it with more than two fetuses. If the

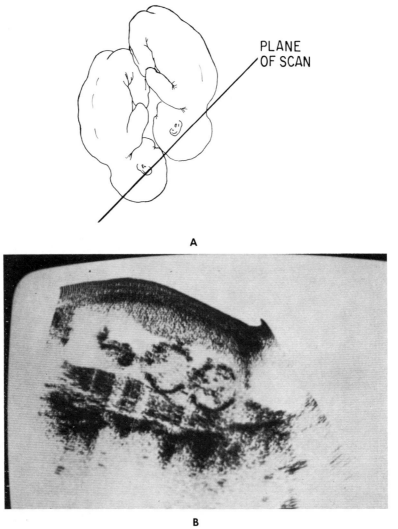

A

B

Figure 10–15. Both fetal heads must be shown on the same scan to verify a diagnosis of twins. A, A diagrammatic representation of the scan plane needed to diagnose twins. B, A scan through the plane shown in A: both fetal heads are seen.

patient seems too large for dates, she may well have a multiple gestation, and the ultrasonographer has to be on guard. Usually scanning carefully with the standard routine will produce whatever data are needed to make the diagnosis. If we have identified more than one fetus, we like to record both fetal heads in a single scan by angling the scanner arm as necessary to do this (Fig. 10–15). Sometimes it can be difficult to tell whether we are dealing with a fetal head or thorax. Visualization of the heart beat will allow us to differentiate between these two; and that leads us to our next topic, the recognition and recording of the fetal heart beat.

FETAL HEART BEAT

We come now to another instance when the availability of bi-stable recording is a great help. Frequently, while scanning over the trunk of the baby, a tiny moving echo will appear as a squiggly line (Fig. 10–16). By holding the transducer stationary at the point where this is observed and changing gain settings so that the image can be used on the bi-stable screen, a moving echo can be recognized bouncing up and down. Sometimes it takes a bit of angling of the transducer to bring the echo into view clearly. This moving echo is produced by the heart, usually the ventricular wall. Recording this motion is simply

done by switching the machine to the M-mode. If your scanner has depth markers it is usually a help to position the marker below the point where the movement is seen before changing over to M-mode so that you can tell where the echo should be if it is not visible as the sweep moves across the scope. We adjust the speed of the sweep so that we can record for at least three seconds (Fig. 10–17). We do not recommend this technique as the standard ultrasonic means of confirming the fetal heart beat; obviously using a Doppler instrument is much easier and faster. We want to stress that recording the fetal heart beat with the B-scanner is primarily an aid in differentiating the fetal trunk from the head to decide about fetal presentation and the possibility of multiple gestation. (There are rare occasions where for one reason or another a fetal heart beat cannot be detected with the Doppler instrument; if B-mode scanning can visualize the heart beat in such a case, the viability of the pregnancy can be confirmed.)

OTHER OBSERVATIONS OF THE FETUS

One of the great ultrasound games is the demonstration of fetal anatomy, normal and abnormal. As the use of real-time scanners in which motion is more easily observed becomes more prevalent, evaluation of the

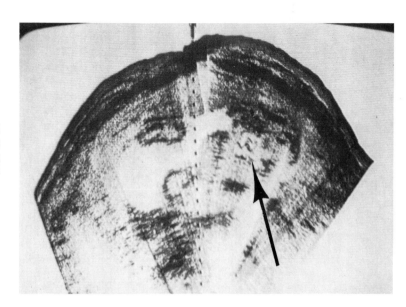

Figure 10–16. The fetal heart is often seen as a wiggly structure *(arrow)* on scans through the fetal thorax.

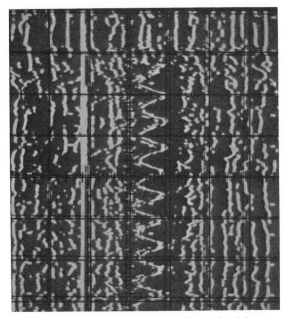

Figure 10–17. The motion of the fetal heart can be documented in M-mode (cf. Figure 3–9). The sawtooth appearance is due to the motion of the ventricular walls.

fetus will move out of the realm of speculation and become a matter of routine. For the moment, however, there are some things about the fetus which we can define even now, and with practice one becomes quite adept at this. For instance, we can usually recognize gross abnormalities of the head such as anencephaly, hydrocephalus, collapse of the calvarium because of fetal death, or edema of the scalp. We can appreciate the presence of ascites in the belly of a baby, and even abnormal kidneys have been seen because of their large size or echo-free dilated collecting systems. Sometimes, we can determine sex (particularly if the baby is a male) by identifying male external genitalia (Fig. 10–18). (*Proceed with caution department:* It is probably wise not to tell the mother what you have decided regarding the sex of her child, because this can be somewhat unsettling. Certainly with the present state of our capability to determine the sex of the fetus with conventional B-mode scanning, we would not advise any action be taken on the ultrasound diagnosis alone. There are instances where a diagnosis of sex is quite important—for instance, when dealing with families in which there is a history of certain familial diseases such as hemophilia. If definitive determination of fetal sex is required, it is still necessary to depend upon chromosomal analysis.)

AMNIOCENTESIS

One of the obstetrical procedures you will be called upon to support rather frequently is amniocentesis. Examination of the amniotic fluid is becoming increasingly common for a variety of reasons. Genetic counseling and evaluation of fetal maturity are probably the most common. Sometimes, however, it is necessary to inject medication into the gestational sac rather than to remove fluid (for instance, when performing a prostaglandin-induced abortion). You may therefore be dealing with a relatively early (12 to 16 weeks) gestation. Actually, there is no trick to this; what one looks for is the echo-free zone indicating the presence of a pool of amniotic fluid into which a needle can be reliably introduced. We want to avoid spearing the fetus; and if we can manage it, it is best to avoid the

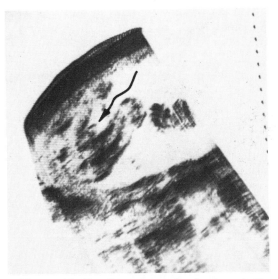

Figure 10–18. Sometimes the fetal genitalia can be identified between the thighs, enabling the ultrasonographer to predict the baby's sex. This is a scan of a baby boy *(arrow)*. Figure 10–12A shows a baby girl.

MARY HITCHCOCK MEMORIAL HOSPITAL
DEPARTMENT OF RADIOLOGY
REPORT OF ULTRASOUND EXAMINATION

Stark, Molly
Bennington, Vt.
02 17 75-3

REFERRING PHYSICIAN:
Dr. N. Smith,
Hanover, N.H.

Date of exam: *4/1/76*

HISTORY: EDC: *6/15/76*   HOW CALCULATED:
                                 Physical exam_____
REASON FOR EXAM: Menstrual History __✓__ LMP *9/8/75*

  Gestational age (Placental localization) Intrauterine growth retardation

  Amniocentesis   Multiple pregnancy (Bleeding) Fetal demise

ULTRASOUND FINDINGS:

  I.   GESTATION: (Single)
                  Multiple (If multiple, data on this page refers to baby
                            number____of____.)

  II. PRESENTATION:
          (Cephalic) Breech   Transverse (back up)   Transverse (back down)

  III. PLACENTAL LOCALIZATION:
          (Anterior) Posterior   Left lateral (Right lateral)   fundal

          Complete praevia (Marginal praevia)

          Comments: *This placenta should "migrate" to*
          permit vaginal delivery.

  IV. PLACENTAL TEXTURE: (Homogeneous)   Inhomogeneous

  V.   GESTATIONAL AGE:
          Diameter of gestational sac_____cm. or bi-parietal diameter *7.4* cm.
          Age based on measurement *29* weeks.

  VI. FETAL SEX: Male   Female (Undertermined)

  VII. Comments:

                                    RADIOLOGIST _____

Figure 10–19.   Both we and our obstetricians like a simplified "circle-the-right-answer" or "fill-in-the-blank" type of report form for obstetrical examinations.

placenta. The objective is to obtain clear fluid, uncontaminated by blood.

In preparation for amniocentesis we scan the uterus both longitudinally and transversely, looking for the most convincing collection of fluid and then mark on the abdomen where the puncture will be most likely to be successful. It usually works out that the space where the fetal small parts lie is the best target. If in order to enter that space it is necessary to go through the placenta, one can generally do this without difficulty; but it is preferable to avoid the middle where the large umbilical blood vessels are usually located. The placenta should never be punctured in an Rh negative mother. (*Reminder:* The centimeter marker should be flashed onto the screen so that the depth at which the fluid will be found can be measured.)

Amniocentesis obviously requires a sterile tray with drapes, needles, syringes, etc.; and the skin must have a sterile prep. This equipment should be assembled into a pack for sterilization after you have gone over the needs with the individual who will do the tap; we will not attempt to list them further for you here. Again, introducing the needle is an invasive procedure and as such should be preserved for the physician.

It is always better to do an amniocentesis on the same table in the ultrasound lab where the scanning has been performed rather than have the patient hike back to the obstetrical clinic or floor to have the puncture done there. The likelihood that the fetus will move and upset the relationship demonstrated on the scan is very great if the patient gets off the table; and you are probably destined to frustratingly unsuccessful taps if you allow the patient to move after localizing the puncture site.

REPORT OF OBSTETRICAL EXAMINATION

We have found it helpful to report obstetrical ultrasound examinations on a preprinted, circle-the-right-answer or fill-in-the-blank form (Fig. 10–19). This is really not a big deal; we have one of our departmental secretaries type out the original form which is then photocopied. (We change the format rather frequently, so we have not had it printed up.) We review the scans while the patient is still in the ultrasound lab and immediately fill out the form so that, when the patient leaves the department, the report is complete and ready for distribution.

A glance at the report form will help fix in your mind the various aspects of the obstetrical examination which are important to note and emphasize what should be reported. The top sections contain patient identification information and historical data—Mickey Mouse stuff that is, nonetheless, important. Next we count babies and report the number found. We locate the placenta. Then we describe how each fetus is positioned, not in elaborate detail, just what part is presenting at the cervix. Next comes our estimate of fetal age, an important piece of information almost always. Finally, we may comment on fetal sex and any other observation about the baby or the uterus we may have made. Usually, we acquire all of this information on every obstetrical ultrasound we do. It may not be necessary, however, to make an elaborate report if the question asked is very specific, such as estimation of gestational age. Because locating the fetal head to determine fetal age will almost always provide the other data, it seems only sensible to report it.

Chapter 11

MISCELLANEOUS EXAMINATIONS

As your expertise (and your fame) in scanning increases, it is inevitable that you will be approached to perform some more unusual examinations. This usually comes up indirectly; a physician will casually ask you, "Say, is this ultrasound stuff any good for testicular masses?" Or "pain in the knee," or "lumps on the back," and so on. Great ultrasound boosters that we are, we always answer this with either, "Why, of course!" or, if we have no idea whatsoever, "Probably, but I'm not sure. Why don't you send the patient over and I'll see what I can do." We do not always succeed in obtaining clinically useful information, of course; but it is fun to try and one never knows what will be learned. Because ultrasound is neither harmful nor unpleasant for the patient, it is worthwhile to try the study even if it is a long shot. In this chapter we shall discuss briefly some less common examinations which we have been called on to perform and describe our approach to them.

THYROID

It is misleading to place thyroid examinations in the "less common" category, inasmuch as B-mode scanning of the thyroid is a well-established procedure. It is not at all infrequent that a patient with a thyroid mass or enlargement will be sent to the ultrasound laboratory for evaluation; this topic does not fit in well any place else in the text, however, and so we have chosen to discuss it here.

The most common question which occurs is whether a palpable thyroid mass (always called a "nodule" for some reason) is cystic or solid. Usually these patients will already have had an isotope scan of the thyroid, and the suspicious area will have

failed to take up the agent (making it a so-called "cold" nodule). Although many thyroid tumors are "cold," so are benign thyroid cysts; and it is very helpful to the clinician to know if this potentially dangerous mass is only a simple thyroid cyst. This is where ultrasound comes in: if the ultrasound examination shows a cystic structure, a simple needle aspiration can be performed to confirm the diagnosis and no further evaluation may be necessary. On the other hand, if the ultrasound shows a solid mass, the clinician will want to investigate it more fully. By using any of the commercially available scanners it should be possible to make this distinction quite accurately in the great majority of patients. (*Somewhere-in-the-future department:* Although there are scattered reports in the literature which indicate it may be possible to distinguish benign from malignant solid thyroid masses on the basis of the ultrasound echo pattern alone, we do not feel that this is feasible at the present time, using commercially available equipment. Certainly we have not had much success in doing this and, in talking with other ultrasonographers from around this country and the world, we learn that most laboratories have had the same experience. This does not mean that such diagnoses are impossible, and in a few years technical advances in transducer and scanner design may permit this to be done routinely.) In addition to evaluating the nature of a thyroid mass, ultrasound can outline the boundaries of the gland and give an accurate estimation of its size and shape. Some physicians use the ultrasound examination to follow the effects of their treatment of goiters and thyroiditis.

It is not difficult to scan the thyroid if the patient is properly positioned so that the gland is easily accessible. We have had the most success with the patient in the supine position, with a bulky pillow under the upper thorax so that the head hangs over the back of the pillow and the neck is extended. The thyroid is then pulled up from the manubrium and thrust forward (Fig. 11–1). We have the patient remove shirt, sweater, or blouse so that we will not have to worry about spilling oil.

There is some controversy as to whether it is better to use contact scanning (that is, the transducer in direct *contact* with the patient's skin) or water bath coupled scanning. A case can be made for either method. Contact scanning is certainly easier and, if you have a delicate touch, can give perfectly satisfactory results. Since the thyroid is soft and close to the skin surface you must be very careful not to displace or distort it with the transducer. Because the gland is so superficial there can also be problems with resolution. It is difficult to focus a transducer closer than 2 centimeters from its face; and this means that portions of the gland are usually located in a zone of relatively poor focus where the resolution is decreased. If the transducer is set off a few centimeters in a water bath, however, the gland can be examined by using the best focus of the sound beam, with some improvement in resolution. Also, the use of a water bath eliminates the problem of distortion of the thyroid by transducer contact. Water bath scanning is not without its problems, however: the water bath is awkward to set up and position over the patient; it is difficult to get good contact between the bath and the skin (all air must be excluded); and only limited scanning motion is possible since the electric parts of the transducer and arm must not come in contact with the water. An alternative method of water bath coupling is to use a closed water bag which is simply placed over the patient's neck; the transducer is then scanned across the bag. A surgical glove filled with water can be used for this. Although closed water bags eliminate the problem of the transducer coming in contact with the water, they usually require considerable manipulation to be kept in good contact with the patient's skin and often contain trapped air bubbles which interfere with the scan. We have used all of these methods, but favor contact scanning for most cases. (If you are interested in water bath scans there is a reference in the bibliography which shows how to construct a simple water bath at very low cost.)

Because the thyroid is so close to the skin surface and is usually less than 2 centimeters thick, it is possible to use a 5 MHz transducer, which will give some improvement in resolution over the lower frequencies. (This improvement is mainly in lateral resolution, you will remember.) We think that a transducer with a small face (6 mm diameter) produces a better picture than one with a larger (13 mm) face. It is difficult to scan with the small transducer,

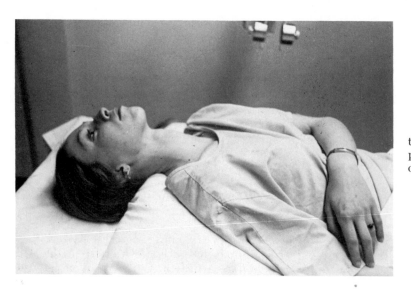

Figure 11–1. It is easiest to scan the thyroid when the patient's neck is extended over a pillow.

however; the tip of the transducer gets caught easily on the skin and tends to dig into and distort the gland. A newer transducer is available which has a large, blunt tip which encases the 6 mm transducer face, and this adaptation makes contact scanning much easier.

A coordinate system is often unnecessary for thyroid scans because the clinical question is usually whether a specific nodule is cystic or solid. Sometimes it will be necessary to scan the entire gland, and in those situations it is useful to have a labeling system to keep the pictures in proper sequence. For longitudinal sections the same coordinates as the abdomen are appropriate (see Chapter 6 for more details of this system). Transverse sections require a different "O" line, however; the iliac crests are too far away to be useful as a reference point. Any bony landmark in the area will do; we use the sternal notch. As always, displacements which are toward the patient's head are considered positive and those toward the feet negative. When label-

ing transverse sections of the thyroid we use an "M" (signifying *manubrium*) instead of the "C" (for *crests*) which we used in the abdomen (Fig. 11–2).

The same general scanning techniques apply here as in the abdomen: proper gain and TCG, single pass scans, and enough sections to answer the clinical question which has been raised. This is one instance in which it is helpful to use the 1:1 scale, and this requires a really steady hand to produce a technically satisfactory scan. The most common clinical question is whether a mass is solid or cystic; and we can apply the same principles for making this distinction that we did in the kidney or abdomen (Fig. 11–3).

TESTICLE

As with the thyroid the usual indication for examining the testicle is to determine whether a mass is solid or cystic. Cystic masses are usually benign hydroceles or spermatoceles, whereas solid masses are usually malignant tumors. There is very little written about testicle scanning and so you are best advised to use your own imagination and improvise. If the mass is large and easily palpated, probably the easiest approach is to simply grab it with one hand (gently, of course) and stabilize it while making a contact scan with the other hand. If the mass is too small to be immobilized this way, it may be necessary to use a water bath to avoid distorting the area while scanning. It can be a tricky business to support the testicle properly so that good contact can be made with a water bath, and we recommend that you make considerable effort to obtain a contact scan. Because of the relatively small size of most testicular masses, a 5 MHz transducer is used; some masses are surprisingly large, however, and will require a 3.5 MHz or 2.25 MHz transducer for adequate penetration. Clearly, a coordinate system is out of the question with such a moveable organ.

Examples of solid and cystic testicular masses are shown in Figure 11–4. Torsion of the testicle is an uncommon condition which has been diagnosed by using a Doppler apparatus but we have no knowledge of anyone using B-mode scanning in this situation.

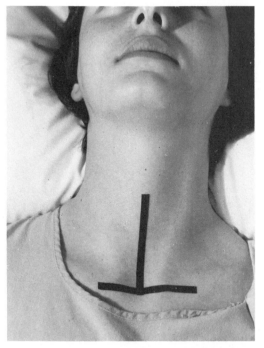

Figure 11–2. The midline is used as the reference plane for longitudinal scans of the thyroid. Transverse scans are labeled relative to the line through the sternal notch, however. This is the "M,0" plane, the M standing for manubrium.

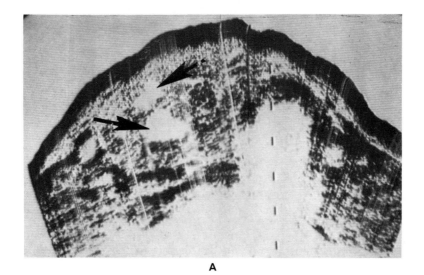

A

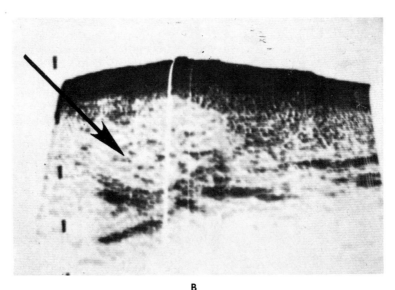

B

Figure 11–3. It is possible to tell whether a thyroid nodule is cystic or solid by using B-mode ultrasound.

A, A transverse section through a large right lobe of the thyroid, showing two small cysts *(arrows)*.

B, Longitudinal scan through a palpable thyroid nodule *(arrow)*. Low level echoes indicate a solid mass.

EXTREMITIES

Any lump or bump on the surface of the body is fair game for the transducer. Most of the time the ultrasound scan will show a solid tissue mass rather than a fluid-filled area and a biopsy or excision will be done. Nevertheless, occasionally the scan will reveal a cystic structure such as a hematoma or abscess. About the only advice we can give concerning these scans is to use the highest frequency transducer possible and be very careful not to cause distortion while scanning. There is nothing like a lump in an unusual or inaccessible location to bring out your true ingenuity.

One area where masses are fairly common is the popliteal fossa—the area behind the knee. By far the greatest number of these are so-called Baker's cysts, a benign outpouching of the synovium of the knee joint. Ultrasound can document the cystic

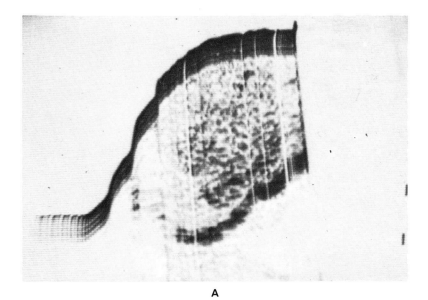

A

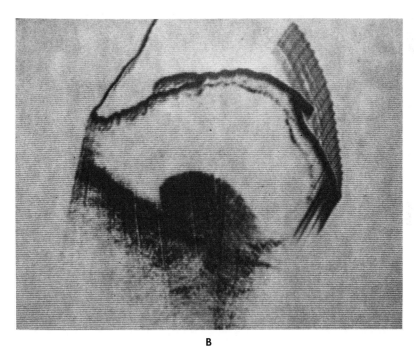

B

Figure 11-4. Ultrasound can determine whether a testicular mass is solid or cystic.
A, A solid tumor of the testicle (seminoma).
B, A large hydrocele. (Courtesy of Dr. J. H. McCutcheon.)

nature of these masses, determine their size, and follow their progression (Fig. 11–5). In these cases it is important to identify the popliteal artery and be certain that it is normal because popliteal artery aneurysm is always a differential diagnostic possibility. Generally we scan longitudinally only, following the long axis of the leg. It is important to scan the posterior surface behind the knee into the upper calf at relatively close (0.5 cm.) intervals so as to be able to identify the artery.

If your laboratory has a Doppler unit, you can use it to evaluate the veins of the leg for blood clots. Although the accuracy of Doppler venography is disputed, there are some investigators who feel it is valuable as a screening examination in patients

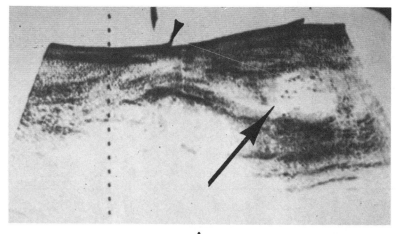

A

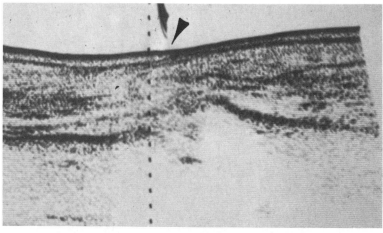

B

Figure 11–5. Ultrasound is useful in deciding if soft tissue masses are fluid-filled or solid.

A, A longitudinal scan of the popliteal fossa and calf, showing a Baker's cyst *(arrow)*. The patient is supine and the scan was done along the midline of the leg. The arrowhead at top points to the back of the popliteal fossa.

B, Scan of the same area several weeks later; the cyst has resolved.

suspected of thrombophlebitis or phlebothrombosis. A few years ago we performed this examination for a short period of time: the results were not useful clinically, however, and so we discontinued the procedure. We shall not discuss this technique but have included a reference in the bibliography for those who would like to pursue it further.

CHEST

Ultrasound has limited utility in the chest (except for evaluation of the heart, of course) because there is always so much air present. (The competition is tough here too; the chest film is one of the best X-ray examinations there is for detecting pathologic conditions.) A few years back there was some enthusiasm for using ultrasound to detect early pulmonary infarctions but this has not proved useful in clinical practice. We can detect pleural effusions, of course, since it is an easy matter to find an echoless area of fluid underneath the chest wall. There is very little need for this, however, because almost all pleural effusions can be clearly identified on the chest X-ray. Sometimes, when there is old pleural scarring, the fluid will be loculated with an atypical X-ray appearance, and you may be called on to clarify the situation. On other occasions the physician may be having difficulty performing a thoracentesis and will ask you to localize a fluid collection for him. We do this by having the patient sit backwards in an armless chair and rest his arms and chin on the chair back. The scanning arm is brought over the patient's shoulder and sector scans are performed between the ribs until an area of fluid is found. This point is then marked on the skin to localize the best spot for needle entry (Fig. 11–6). If possible, the thoracentesis should be done in the ultrasound room, before the patient changes his position (and perhaps the position of the fluid).

Although the lung cannot be examined with ultrasound, the chest wall can. Many radiotherapists like to evaluate the chest wall thickness when they prepare treatment plans involving radiation to the chest. B-mode ultrasound scans can be used for this purpose, and, if your radiotherapist is interested, you may have the opportunity to scan some chest walls. In this case, you should tailor your examination to provide the information the therapist is seeking.

We have not found B-mode scanning useful for mediastinal masses. There are two reasons for this: first, because of overlying lung or bone there is no acoustic window and it is, therefore, usually impossible to see the mediastinum. Second, the normal mediastinum is full of "cysts" (the great arteries and veins) and in the face of these, it is often hard to differentiate an abnormal mass from normal anatomic structures. If a mass is huge and abuts the chest wall, of course it can be assessed with ultrasound and it can at least be determined whether it is cystic or solid.

BREAST

There is considerable interest in ultrasound examination of the breast, not only because breast disease is so common but also because there has been some concern raised as to the possible harmful effects of X-ray mammograms (we will not go into the validity of these concerns here). Several ultrasound laboratories have been working on this problem and have had

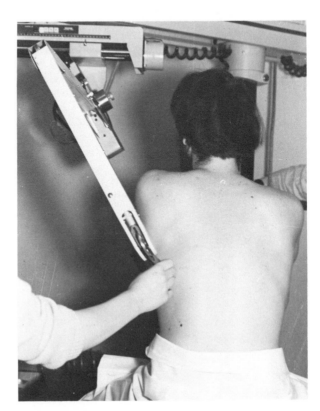

Figure 11–6. Localizing pleural effusions for thoracentesis is best done with the patient sitting in an armless chair.

some encouraging results using special scanning equipment. Unfortunately, this work is still in the investigational stage and, at the present time, ultrasound has very little use in the routine evaluation of breast disease. Why should this be so? After all, there is no gas or bone to cause artifacts and the breast is quite accessible for examination; ultrasound should be great here.

Well, first there is the problem of coupling. As we know, the breast is a delightfully malleable organ and, as such, is easily distorted by the transducer during contact scanning. When the underlying tissue is moved, the interfaces move and the picture becomes meaningless. For this reason, it is impossible to perform an adequate contact scan of the breast and some type of water bath coupling is required. The simple water bath which is used for the thyroid is neither large nor stable enough to encompass a breast; a large, specially constructed bath is needed. There is no easy way to apply a water bath to the breast; if the bath is simply lowered over it, the tissue is flattened out and compressed, or displaced into the axilla. Ideally, the breast should be free-floating in the water but this involves a complicated sealing operation to prevent leaking. Some researchers have suspended the patient over the water with the breast hanging down and scanned from underneath! There is no easy answer; and, until the problem of coupling is solved, breast scanning will not become a routine procedure.

Another serious problem is resolution. X-ray mammography has extremely fine resolution—an order of magnitude better than ultrasound can ever hope to provide (because of the physical limitations we examined in Chapter 1). X-ray mammography can be a very accurate method of detecting small breast cancers, but this accuracy is dependent in large part on the extremely high resolution of the mammogram—the anatomic criteria used for differentiating benign and malignant masses often require resolution of 0.1 mm. It would appear that since ultrasound cannot approach this resolution, it will not be possible for the ultrasound scan, using only the parameters of echo position and amplitude, to compete seriously with the mammogram. It is quite possible that, by simultaneously measuring several other ultrasonic parameters, a highly specific identification of tissue can be made without the necessity for resolution greater than 1 mm. But all this is in the future; at present there are no commercially available scanners which can perform an adequate breast examination.

Of course, if there is a large, palpable breast mass—at least 2 centimeters in diameter and usually much larger—we can treat it like any lump on the skin and scan it to see if it is cystic or solid. If it is cystic, it can be aspirated for diagnosis; if solid, it can be excised. We are not certain how useful this ultrasound information is to the overall management of the patient. Almost all breast masses this size will have either excision biopsy or aspiration anyway, regardless of the ultrasound findings. It probably comes down to your local surgeon's general approach to breast masses. He may wish to know if a palpable mass is cystic before proceeding: if so, then the ultrasound scan is a useful examination. If he does not care about this information, the scan is a waste of time. We do not mean to be pessimistic when asked about ultrasound and the breast—in a few years technologic developments may make it the procedure of choice; in the meantime, we try to do what we can.

Chapter 12

BI-STABLE SCANNING

The era of bi-stable scanning is rapidly receding in the distance, outpaced by the glamor and utility of gray scale. In less than two years' time it has gone from the status of standard of the art to a forgotten relic. Why then, a chapter on bi-stable technique? Well, like that classic of the automobile world, the '57 Chevy, it may be outmoded but it still is a good technique and, in some situations, has much to offer. Actually, there is very little difference in the basic sounder between gray-scale and bistable machines; only the display format differs. You will read in some articles that gray scale offers "more information," "much more," "8 times more"—or some such nonsense—than bi-stable scans. This simply isn't true! The same information is available with both techniques—it is just much more difficult to extract with a bi-stable instrument. Virtually all the diagnostic criteria in use today were formulated on bistable scanners. We are not advocating overthrow of gray scale; on the contrary, we believe that the introduction of commercial gray-scale scanners represented the turning point in the widespread acceptance of diagnostic ultrasound. The ease and speed of scanning with these machines has made ultrasound available to the community hospital and private office as well as the medical center. There is no question that gray scale should be the basis for the overwhelming majority of examinations. Nonetheless, there are a few scanning situations where the bi-stable mode has distinct advantages, and if your scanner has bi-stable capability, we think you will find it advantageous to use it on occasion.

Before proceeding we should clarify what we mean by the term "bi-stable." Strictly defined it means "existing in two states" or, from the ultrasonic point of view, "having only two shades—black and white." This is too broad a definition for us. When we speak of bi-stable we mean a display mode which utilizes a **storage oscilloscope** rather than a scan converter–TV display format. The oscilloscope has two distinct advantages over a TV format: first, it has sharper definition of edges or dot margins (assuming a large, high quality scope) and second (and most important), it permits continuous visualization of the ultrasound beam—that is, it permits the ultrasonographer to observe the echoes even when they are not being written on the storage target. It is clear that what most manufacturers are calling bi-stable mode today is really just high contrast gray scale and, as such, has little or no advantage over the regular gray scale. If the output is a TV monitor, it is not bi-stable by our definition. While this may seem like nit-picking it actually is an important distinction, as we shall see.

SCANNING TECHNIQUE

In Chapters 3 and 6 we briefly mentioned "outlining," the technique used for bistable scanning. Because there is no way to distinguish between the amplitude of echoes, bi-stable scans cannot utilize tissue texture to arrive at a diagnosis. If too many echoes are received, the entire image becomes white and little diagnostic information is available. To get around this problem, bi-stable scans are performed at a much lower gain than gray-scale scans and only the loudest echoes are received. In practice these are usually the loud, specular echoes from the capsule of organs and the boundaries of vessels and masses. Using these loud echoes, an outline map of the internal anatomy is made: organs and masses are identified by their outline rather than their internal texture. Figure 12–1 shows a bi-stable scan of the upper abdomen where the outline of various organs and vessels is quite clear. Notice that these boundaries can be identified very precisely on the bi-stable scan; this is because of the sharper edge resolution of the oscilloscope display and the fact that the scan is performed at low gain. Because of this precise echo localization, bi-stable scans are very useful when accurate measurements are needed—measuring a biparietal diameter in a fetus, for example.

Now, since we are interested primarily in specular echoes which are angle-dependent (remember, in Chapter 1, we saw that the strength of a specular echo depends upon the angle at which the ultrasound beam strikes the interface), we want to move the transducer so that the sound beam hits the interfaces from as many angles as possible. The best way to accom-

plish this is with compound scanning (Fig. 6–8). Because we are not preserving amplitude information, we are not concerned with having the beam pass over an interface more than once; we are now trying to find where the interface is located, and any technique which gives the echo a better chance of being recorded is useful. For most bi-stable scans, therefore, we should use a compound scanning motion. going back and forth across the patient and "painting in" the outline of the internal anatomy. Of course, artifacts are present with bi-stable as well as gray scale, so we want to keep the transducer over an acoustic window as much as possible. We still will not scan over bowel or ribs (although we will probably make a sector in every interspace). Because we are using lower gain, however, artifacts will not be as much a problem with bi-stable as they are with gray scale.

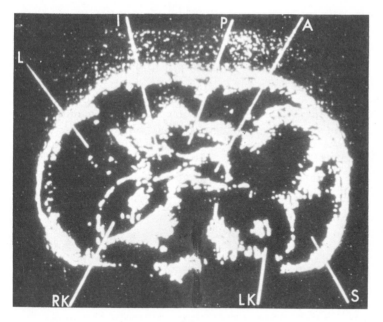

Figure 12–1. Internal anatomy is recognized by the outline of organs and masses when scanning with a bi-stable display. This is a picture of a transverse scan of the normal upper abdomen. L = liver. I = inferior vena cava. P = portal vein. A = aorta. S = spleen. LK = left kidney. RK = right kidney. (Courtesy of Dr. H. H. Holm.)

Figure 12–2. The continuously variable gain technique is used to obtain echo amplitude information in bi-stable scans.

A, The scan is started at very low gain so that only the loudest echoes are recorded.

B, *Without erasing the image* the scan is repeated with the gain increased; this adds the middle intensity echoes.

C, *Without erasing the image* the scan is again repeated at still higher gain; the weakest echoes are now added to the picture. Notice that the final picture is not very useful: it is the order in which the echoes appear that is important.

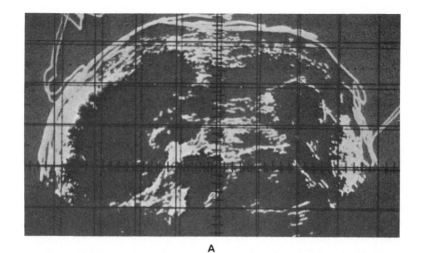

A

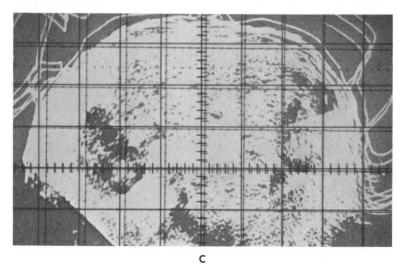

B

C

Figure 12–2. See legend on the opposite page.

CONTINUOUSLY VARIABLE GAIN TECHNIQUE

Even though amplitude data cannot be recorded directly on a storage oscilloscope, the information is still available and can be obtained by using the continuously variable gain technique. As the name suggests, this involves changing the gain continuously while the scan is being performed. We start with the gain very low, so that only the loudest echoes will be recorded on the screen, and "paint in" an outline image. This will represent the strongest echoes in the patient—those that would appear in the darkest shade of gray. Once we have this image in mind we increase the gain slightly and paint over the picture once again, adding the next loudest echoes. We do not erase the image between passes, instead we just keep painting over the picture while slowly increasing the gain; this will permit us to gradually fill in our outline image with internal echoes. By observing when specific echoes appear we can get some idea as to their amplitude. This is illustrated in Figure 12–2.

This continuously variable gain technique is somewhat analogous to the way an artist paints a picture; he starts by sketching in an outline of the picture, then adds the basic coloring and structure to his sketch, and finally puts in the fine details and subtle shading. Of course, the final result is quite different. The artist will have a complete and detailed picture when he is finished while our bi-stable ultrasound image will be almost totally white and have very little information. This illustrates a basic difference between bi-stable and gray-scale scanning; in bi-stable it is the way in which the image is built up, the order in which echoes appear on the screen as the gain is increased, which is important rather than the final picture. In fact the final bi-stable picture is relatively worthless, because there is no way of knowing the relationships between the strengths of the echoes. This undoubtedly was responsible for the limited enthusiasm for B-mode ultrasound before the introduction of gray scale; in those days it was difficult to produce an image which actually looked like recognizable anatomy and this made people skeptical. If you took a bi-stable picture (which often looked like the art work of a pre–nursery school student) to a surgeon and told him that the patient had an adrenal mass he would smile patiently, politely agree that "this certainly is an interesting new thing, this ultrasound," and go away thinking that you must be on LSD if you are able to see anything in the mess of chicken scratches on that picture. What the surgeon could not appreciate, of course, was that you had actually seen the adrenal mass as it was outlined and then filled in with echoes during the scanning process. There is no really satisfactory way of conveying this process to someone who was not present when the scan was actually being performed. The best that we can do is to make two or three photographs of each image, at low, medium, and high gain for example, to try to document the formation as it appeared on the screen (Fig. 12–3).

Bi-stable scanning, then, is analogous to X-ray fluoroscopy: the information is collected and the diagnostic decision made during the actual scanning procedure. It is imperative, therefore, that the person who has the responsibility for reading the scan also be the person who performs the scan; the hard copy pictures cannot stand by themselves.

SINGLE PASS SCANNING

The single pass scan technique, the mainstay of gray scale, is also useful in bi-stable, providing the ultrasonographer already has a good idea of what he is looking for. If a mass has been identified by the continuously variable gain scan, it is useful to make a few single pass scans of it to get the maximum resolution and best definition. Figure 12–4 shows how this can be applied to the measurement of a biparietal diameter. The fetal head is localized and identified with compound scanning but, when a measurement is to be made, the best definition of the skull can be obtained using a single pass scan. Similarly, we can use compound scanning to evaluate the abdomen and, after an aneurysm has been identified, make one or two single pass pictures to measure its size. In trying to decide if a renal mass is cystic or solid it is very important to evaluate the nature of the back wall—if it is one continuous, smooth line, we can be certain that we are dealing

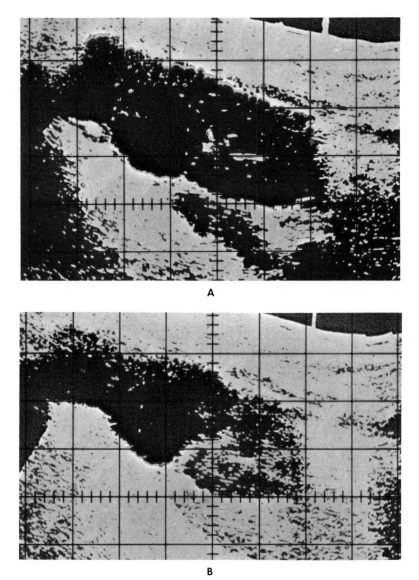

A

B

Figure 12–3. It is necessary to make hard copy photographs at several different gain settings to convey echo amplitude information.

A, A longitudinal scan of the kidney at low gain. There is a cyst in the upper pole.

B, The same section as A but with the gain increased. The echoless nature of the cyst is now apparent but the kidney is obscured.

with a cyst. In order to see this continuous back wall, however, we will have to use a single pass technique.

CURRENT BI-STABLE USES

There are a few scanning situations where we feel that bi-stable technique is preferable to gray scale: (1) when precise measurements are required, such as biparietal diameter or an aneurysm; (2) when motion is being evaluated, such as the fetal heart or aorta; (3) when ultrasonically guided biopsy or amniocentesis is performed; and (4) when there is difficulty in deciding if a mass is cystic or solid.

Because there is extremely sharp edge resolution with an oscilloscope, it is very easy to define the margins of echoes and make precise measurements. Even when a scan converter–TV system is operated as a "bi-stable" display, the exact position of an echo cannot be as accurately seen as with true bi-stable. We use the oscilloscope display for all of our fetal head measurements

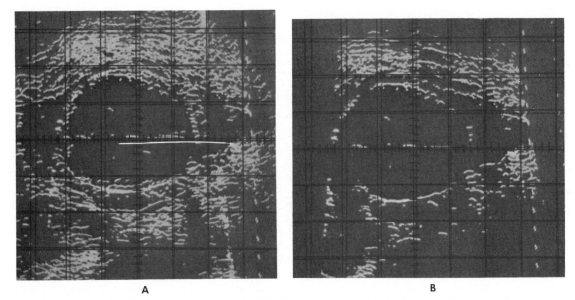

A   B

Figure 12–4. Single pass scanning is useful when precise echo delineation is required.

A, A fetal skull seen with compound scanning. The definition of the skull tables is poor. (Ignore the scratch artifact in the middle of the picture.)

B, The same fetal skull seen with a single pass scan. The edges of the skull are well defined and easy to measure.

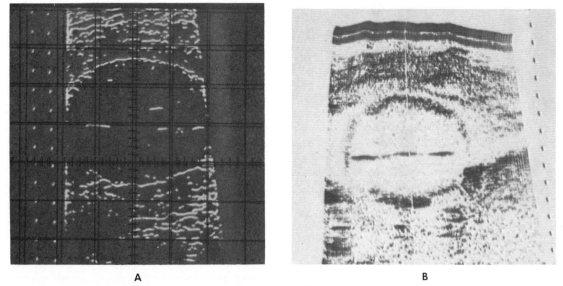

A   B

Figure 12–5. Bi-stable scans have more precise echo boundaries, which make precise measurements easier.

A, A fetal skull in gray scale: the edges of the skull are difficult to measure accurately.

B, The same fetal skull in bi-stable: more precise measurements are possible.

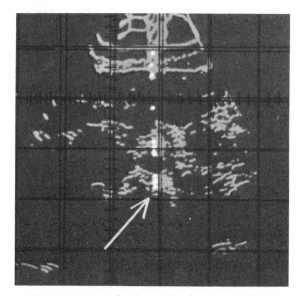

Figure 12-6. The bi-stable display is "live." The actual echoes can always be seen, even when the beam is not writing on the screen. This permits the sound beam to be precisely aimed, as shown in this transverse scan of the upper abdomen. The sound beam *(white arrow)* is aimed through the aorta; the pulsating walls can be easily seen on the screen.

aim the sound beam through each circle and observe what happens to the echoes—if they pulsate then we are looking at the aorta or some other large arterial vessel (Fig. 12-6). We may want to know if a diaphragm is moving or paralyzed; and this, too, can be easily determined by aiming the sound beam through the diaphragm and watching what happens to the echo as the patient breathes.

Ultrasound is the most accurate method of placing a needle in the abdomen for biopsy or amniocentesis but we must be able to tell where the biopsy transducer is aimed during the procedure. This is very easy with bi-stable, but almost impossible with gray scale. (We will discuss biopsy technique in detail in Chapter 13.)

In the great majority of cases it is a simple matter to tell if a renal mass is a cyst, but occasionally some confusion is encountered. When the picture is unclear we have found that the characteristic of the back wall of the mass is the key to the diagnosis. If the back wall is a *continuous, smooth* line we can be certain that we are dealing with a cyst; we have never encountered an abscess or a cystic tumor which had an unbroken, smooth posterior wall (Fig. 12-7). The scan converter–TV display

(Fig. 12-5) and many aneurysm measurements. This sharp edge resolution is also useful in evaluating fetal heart motion in M-mode. Since the fetal heart is so small the echoes from it are often muddled together with a gray-scale display, but can be clearly separated with bi-stable.

Another extremely useful characteristic of the oscilloscope display is that it is "live"—that is, the echoes which are being received are always shown on the screen regardless of any image which is already there. (This is not possible with gray scale because of the problem of overwriting, as discussed in Chapter 3.) This "live" feature enables us to aim the sound beam accurately through any portion of the picture that we desire and see what is happening to the echoes in real time. (Please do not confuse this with real-time scanning which is an entirely different process.) This can be helpful in many ways. For example, we may be having difficulty in deciding which of several small circular echo patterns represents the aorta; it is a simple matter to

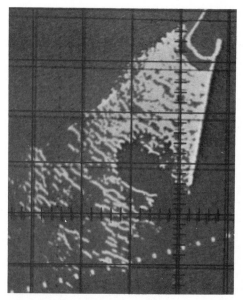

Figure 12-7. Cystic structures have a long, continuous back wall, as illustrated in this picture of a renal cyst. We have never encountered a solid mass which had a *continuous* back wall on the bi-stable scan.

system cannot always reproduce a continuous line because of its inherent construction. (A TV picture is composed of scan lines and it is impossible to record an echo in between these scan lines. For more detail on this see the discussion in Chapter 3.)

PERSPECTIVE

At the risk of being labeled "conservative," "unimaginative," "outmoded," or even—horror of horrors—"backward," we would like to make a plea for the retention of bi-stable capability in new scanners. Admittedly, its usefulness is limited, but it is nonetheless real. In their frantic jump onto the gray-scale bandwagon the equipment manufacturers have abandoned bi-stable—banished might be a more appropriate word—as if it were an embarrassing relic of the past. The "bi-stable" mode on most new machines is nothing more than high contrast gray scale; it still utilizes the scan converter–TV output. If your machine does not have a true bi-stable output (one which utilizes a storage oscilloscope) we recommend that you seriously consider adding it as an optional accessory. The cost is relatively modest and the value quite real. (If you are contemplating biopsies it is essential.) We think that, in the long run, you will find a bi-stable capability at least as useful as many of the other gadgets you could buy, such as an automatic multi-image camera or video tape recorder.

Chapter 13

ULTRASONICALLY GUIDED BIOPSY

Aspiration biopsy of abdominal organs and masses under ultrasonic guidance is one of the older "new" techniques in medicine. The procedure was introduced in Europe in the late 1960's and has been widely used there; however, its acceptance in the United States has been slow. Although the biopsy transducer which is required for the procedure has been available in this country for several years, there has been limited interest in it. It would serve no useful purpose to go into the reasons for the reluctance of American physicians to use this valuable diagnostic technique—let us assume it is due mainly to unfamiliarity with the procedure and its value. This is regrettable because the widespread use of percutaneous biopsy can greatly speed up the diagnostic evaluation of a patient and short-circuit much costly and uninformative testing. We charge all those doing ultrasonography with the responsibility for spreading the word about the procedure and being prepared to perform a biopsy when asked. A biopsy is not limited to suspected renal cysts or tumors but can be applied to any organ or mass which can be identified on the ultrasound scan: suspected abscess, amniocentesis, placenta, dilated renal pelvis, dilated biliary system, pseudocysts, abdominal tumors, etc.—all are areas where the accurate placement of a biopsy needle will yield useful information. The procedure is simple and atraumatic and should be performed *early* in the diagnostic process rather than as a last resort.

EQUIPMENT

The basic tool, of course, is a good quality B-mode scanner. Although we prefer to use gray scale for localizing the mass to be examined by biopsy and for making the appropriate depth measurements, it is necessary to have a bi-stable display (utilizing a storage oscilloscope) for the actual biopsy. A B-mode biopsy transducer is also required. This transducer is exactly the same as a regular transducer with the exception that a narrow hole has been drilled down the axis of the transducer; a needle placed through this hole will be automatically guided along the path of the sound beam. The transducer is also provided with a side arm for attaching it to the scanning arm.

These transducers are commercially available and offer several options such as varying frequencies, center hole dimensions, and lengths. We use two: one is a 3.5 MHz model with an 18 gauge center hole and the other is a 2.25 MHz with a 14 gauge center channel. For most purposes the 3.5 MHz transducer is preferred; but occasionally, when dealing with a deep lesion, we need the extra penetrating power of the lower frequency. The smaller the center hole the better the guidance of the needle. We use a 21 gauge needle for almost all biopsies and, therefore, prefer the 18 gauge center channel. Transducers are also available with removable sides which can be removed from around the needle once it is in place; this is useful if X-ray fluoroscopy or filming is to be performed while the needle is in the patient.

The biopsy transducer must be sterile. This can be accomplished by either gas sterilization or immersion in a liquid antibiotic solution such as 95 per cent alcohol. (The alcohol solution is much more convenient since it can be kept in the ultrasound lab and the transducer is always available; unfortunately the alcohol loosens the glue of some transducers and they may fall apart. If this happens, they can easily be reassembled using a non-soluble glue such as methyacrylate.) A transducer should *never* be heat-sterilized since this may destroy its piezo-electric properties.

(Keep it simple department: In many situations, the target of the biopsy will be so large that use of the biopsy transducer will be unnecessary. A very large renal cyst, amniocentesis, or a large, palpable abdominal mass are all examples of biopsy situations which do not require the use of the biopsy transducer. In these cases, the biopsy procedure is exactly the same as when the transducer is used, with the exception that the steps which involve the special transducer are omitted. We estimate that perhaps 50 to 75 per cent of our biopsies are done without the transducer. If the mass is small, located deep within the abdomen, or is at all difficult to localize precisely, the biopsy transducer should, by all means, be used.)

Any needle can be successfully guided into a mass with a biopsy transducer. We use 21 gauge needles for our work; they are very thin yet are large enough to give a satisfactory cytology specimen in most cases. In over 2000 biopsies of all types of abdominal organs and masses we do not know of any complications involving the use of a needle this small. The needles must be long enough to traverse both the transducer and the tissue overlying the mass; 6-inch and 8-inch lengths are satisfactory. Occasionally the patient's skin is so thick that it is difficult to pass a 21 gauge needle through it and, in these situations, we will use a large needle, 17 or 18 gauge, to traverse the skin and then pass the actual biopsy needle through this "guide needle." You will also need two small, set-screw type needle stops to control the depth of the needle puncture.

When the needle is in place, 10 ml of suction must be applied to get a good specimen: this is most conveniently done with a 12 to 20 ml syringe of either plastic or glass (we prefer glass, but not for any good reason).

There are several minor ancillary items which are necessary. These include: a skin-marking solution for identifying the puncture site, solutions for sterilizing the patient's skin, such as alcohol or Betadine, sterile gloves and drapes, sterile mineral oil for coupling the transducer to the skin, a ruler for measuring needle depth, and cytology fixative and slides or specimen tubes (these can be furnished by your hospital pathology department). You can either make up a small "biopsy kit" containing these items and have it sterilized, as shown in Figure 13–3, or you can use one of the commercially available disposable myelogram trays and add your own needles.

PATIENT PREPARATION

Minimal patient preparation is required; if a mass can be seen by ultrasound scan, it can be subjected to biopsy. (Of course it is important to be certain that we are actually seeing a mass and not just artifacts or bowel. If the presence of the mass has not been confirmed by some other examination such as a physical exam, X-ray, or isotope study, we feel that a second ultrasound scan should be performed after a 48-hour interval to verify the presence of the mass, before proceeding with the biopsy.) We require evidence of a relatively normal blood clotting status—normal qualitative platelets on a blood smear—but nothing else. Although when this procedure was first being performed we had the patients fast, the absence of any complications has caused us to abandon this restriction. An informed consent should be obtained for medico-legal purposes. We do not really believe that this is in any way a dangerous or "experimental" procedure (it is probably safer than an IVP) but, given the current medical liability climate, we agree that "Discretion is the better part of valor."

BIOPSY PROCEDURE

We hope that you like cooking, or at least reading cookbooks, because we are going to describe the actual biopsy procedure in very basic, step-by-step fashion. As with everything we have said it is perfectly permissible to make your own variations; however, we know that if you follow the steps described you will get good results.

Step 1 (Fig. 13–2)

The target of the biopsy (a mass, cyst, amniotic fluid, or whatever) is first located,

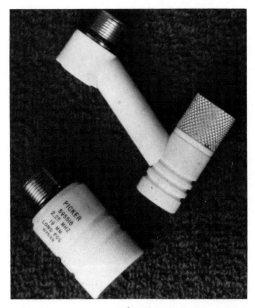

A

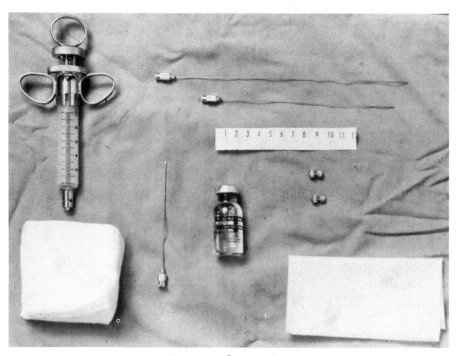

B

Figure 13–1. Little equipment is required for ultrasonically guided biopsy.

A, The biopsy transducer is similar to a standard transducer but has a hole drilled along the axis of the sound beam. This picture shows a standard and a biopsy transducer.

B, A typical biopsy kit containing suction syringe, biopsy needles of varying lengths, a sterile measuring tape, set-screw needle stops, sterile mineral oil, and sterile drapes and sponges.

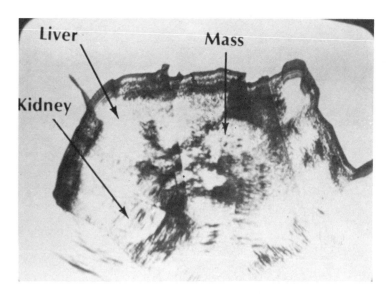

Figure 13-2. Step 1. The mass to be investigated by biopsy is localized with the regular transducer.

using standard B-scan technique and gray scale. In our example in Figure 13–2 the mass is in the pancreas.

Step 2 (Fig. 13–3)

The path for the biopsy is selected. This is usually the shortest distance from the skin to the mass. We try to avoid the liver or other organs if this does not greatly increase the distance; however, we have performed many biopsies through the liver and bowel and there is no problem if these organs are traversed.

Step 3 (Fig. 13–4)

The transducer is moved until it is directly over the selected puncture site on the patient's skin. This is located by observing the main bang echo on the TV monitor. The transducer is removed and the puncture site is marked with an "X" on the skin.

Step 4 (Fig. 13–5)

The distance from the puncture site to the middle of the mass is measured. This

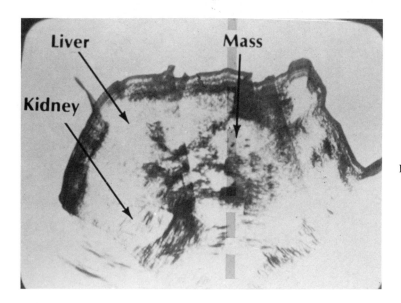

Figure 13-3. Step 2. The path for the biopsy is selected.

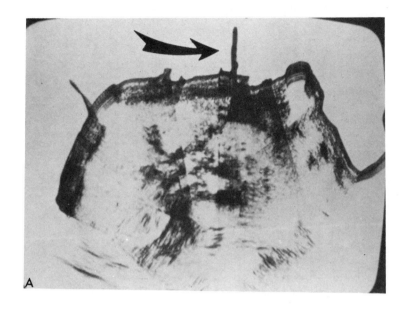

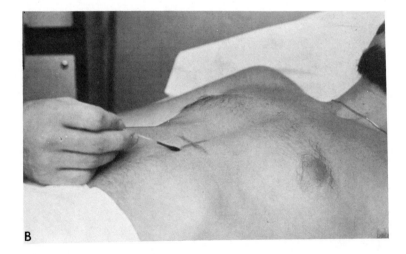

Figure 13–4. Step 3. The needle entry site is marked on the scan *(A)* and the patient's skin *(B)*.

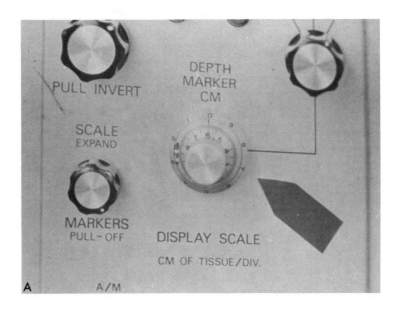

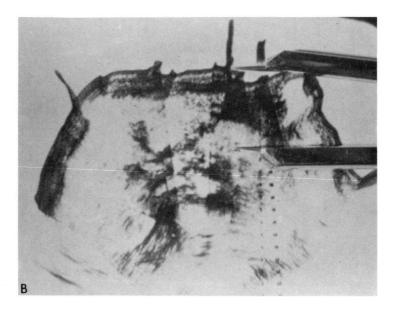

Figure 13–5. Step 4. The depth of needle penetration is measured. This can be done either with a built-in electronic measuring system *(A)* or with calipers on the scan itself *(B)*.

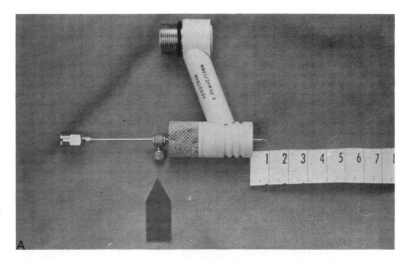

Figure 13–6. Step 5. The depth of needle penetration is set with the needle stops. If an outer guide needle is used it is inserted to a depth of 1 centimeter *(A)*. The biopsy needle is inserted to the depth determined in Step 4 *(B)*.

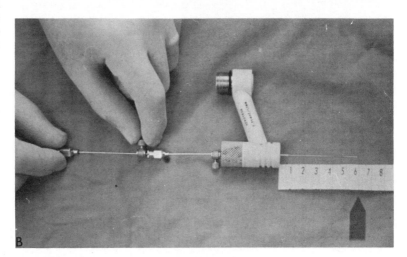

can be done by using the electronic measuring system available in some scanners or by simply measuring the distance on the ultrasound picture with a set of calipers. In our example this distance is 6 centimeters.

Step 5 (Fig. 13–6)

The needle stops are placed on the biopsy needles. Our example shows how this is done if a "guide needle" is used to facilitate passing the small biopsy needle through the skin; however, a guide needle is only necessary if the patient has very thick skin. The guide needle is inserted through the biopsy transducer until its tip projects 1 centimeter past the transducer face and the needle stop is tightened. The biopsy needle is then passed through the guide needle until its tip is the required

distance from the transducer face (this distance was measured in step 4: in our example it is 6 centimeters) and the needle stop is tightened. *Of course, this must all be done with sterile technique.*

Step 6 (Fig. 13–7)

The biopsy transducer is substituted for the regular transducer, with care exercised to keep the biopsy transducer sterile. The side arm of the biopsy transducer must be kept at a right angle (90°) to the scanning plane or the image will be distorted.

Step 7 (Fig. 13–8)

The patient's skin is scrubbed with a sterilizing solution and suitable sterile

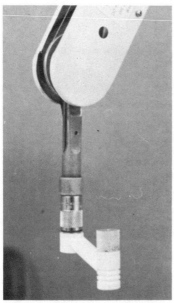

Figure 13-7. Step 6. The biopsy transducer is substituted for the regular transducer. The biopsy transducer must be sterile and the side arm must be at right angles to the scanning plane.

drapes are positioned. Local skin anesthesia can be given but we do not recommend its use: we have found that the anesthesia hurts more than the actual biopsy.

Step 8 (Fig. 13–9)

The scanner is switched to bi-stable display; and, using sterile mineral oil as a coupling agent, the mass is re-scanned with the biopsy transducer. An assistant holds the transducer so that the sound beam passes through the center of the mass.

Step 9 (Fig. 13–10)

The guide needle (if used) is placed through the transducer and skin; and then the biopsy needle, attached to the suction syringe, is quickly thrust through the guide needle to the predetermined depth. Suction of 10 ml is applied (this will take two hands—it is a lot of pressure) and the needle is gently but rapidly moved up and down three or four times within the mass. The suction is released and the biopsy needle withdrawn. The entire operation should take no more than five seconds and the patient should be holding his breath while the biopsy is performed. Sometimes an echo from the needle can actually be seen on the monitor during the biopsy. Although some ultrasonographers get excited about this we do not think it is important. For one thing, we can never be sure that the echo we are seeing corresponds to the needle *tip* as opposed to some other part of the needle, and who cares anyway? We know the position of the needle tip by observing the sound beam since the biopsy transducer is functioning as a bombsight and directing the needle along the path of the sound beam. We have already measured the depth of the mass and placed the needle stop appropriately. So do not waste

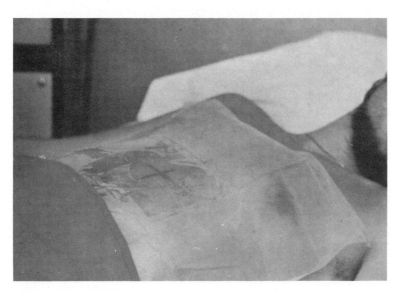

Figure 13-8. Step 7. The patient's skin is sterilized and the area covered with sterile drapes.

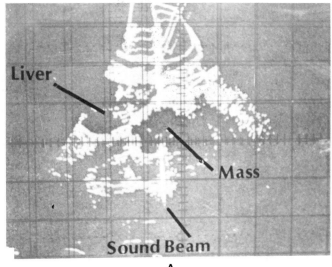

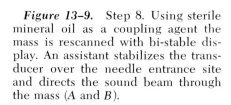

Figure 13–9. Step 8. Using sterile mineral oil as a coupling agent the mass is rescanned with bi-stable display. An assistant stabilizes the transducer over the needle entrance site and directs the sound beam through the mass (*A* and *B*).

A

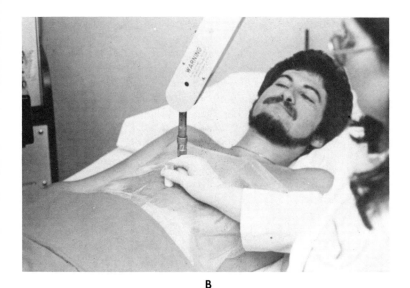

B

Figure 13–10. Step 9. The biopsy needle is rapidly inserted to the predetermined depth, 10 milliliters of suction is applied to the syringe, and the needle moved gently up and down two or three times. Suction is released and the needle is withdrawn.

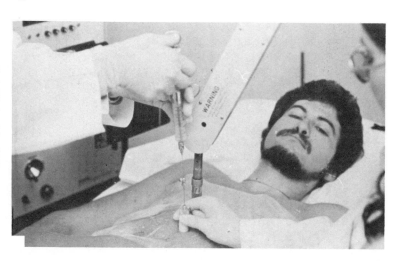

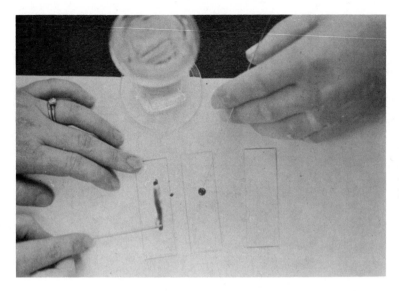

Figure 13–11. Step 10. The specimen is ejected onto slides, smeared, and immediately placed in fixative. Specimen handling varies, depending on the type of biopsy and the laboratory tests to be performed.

your time trying to see the needle on the monitor.

Step 10 (Fig. 13–11)

The specimen is ejected onto slides, smeared, and immediately immersed in fixative. (This depends, of course, on the target of the biopsy. If it is a cyst the fluid is placed in an appropriate specimen tube; if amniotic fluid, special specimen handling may be required; an abscess may require both a smear and a culture tube, etc. Just remember to assemble whatever tubes, slides, or other paraphernalia you will need *before* you begin.) If the mass is solid and cytology is the examination which will be performed, several slides are necessary. Usually only two or three smears may be made from a single needle pass, so make at least three passes of the biopsy needle into the patient (as described in Step 9) and try to have at least 8 to 10 slides for the cytologist. The amount of specimen obtained on any single pass depends on the nature of the mass; pancreatic tumors are often very hard and only scant specimens are obtained while a vascular tumor may yield a copious quantity of material. If the initial needle pass yields little or no specimen, you should be more vigorous with the suction and needle oscillation on subsequent passes. Conversely, if the first specimen is excessively bloody, less suction is needed on the next attempt.

In general, excess blood makes it more difficult for the cytologist to interpret the specimen. Sometimes it is necessary to disconnect the syringe from the needle, fill it with air, and then blow the specimen onto the slide. After the final pass the needle is flushed with a small amount of saline and this also is sent to the laboratory. A good specimen usually permits the cytologist to make a specific diagnosis. In our example (an actual case) the diagnosis was adenocarcinoma of the pancreas (Fig. 13–12).

POST-BIOPSY PRECAUTIONS

Very little follow-up of the patient is required. When these procedures were first performed, elaborate post-biopsy follow-up, including exploratory surgery (which was previously scheduled anyway) was routine. The total absence of any serious side effects in a very large series of patients has caused us to relax considerably our follow-up procedures. In-patients receive hourly vital signs for 4 hours and a hematocrit 24 hours after the procedure. Out-patients are observed in the hospital for four hours and are then discharged, provided they remain within 15 minutes' travel time of the hospital and are capable of contacting a physician should they experience any discomfort. We do not get post-biopsy hematocrits on out-patients. We are even less fretful about patients after amniocentesis. Having monitored fetal heart rate after the

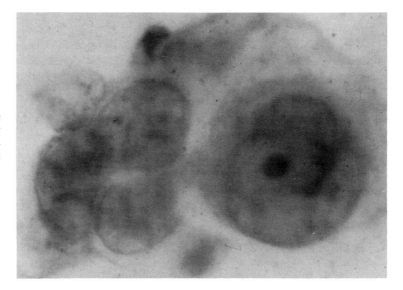

Figure 13–12. Cytologic specimens of excellent quality can be obtained with this procedure. This example shows carcinoma of the pancreas.

tap to determine that it is not changed, we dismiss the patient without further wait. Before a procedure other than amniocentesis is performed on an out-patient basis we screen the patient to make sure that he is capable of recognizing the symptoms of internal bleeding or infection. If we have any doubts as to the patient's competence or reliability we will not do an out-patient biopsy but will schedule an overnight hospital admission. We have not found it necessary to give any analgesics or sedatives either before or after the biopsy.

SAFETY

Sticking needles into people's abdomens sounds like a bad idea—it must be cutting organs up in there and causing trouble, right? Well, we thought so, too, initially; but an extensive experience, primarily in Europe, has demonstrated that this is truly an innocuous procedure. We have personal knowledge of over 2500 biopsies of every abdominal and retroperitoneal organ and in this entire group of patients there has been no mortality or serious morbidity and less than 10 cases of minor morbidity, such as pain lasting for more than an hour, fever, or evidence of bleeding. There have been only three cases of documented hemorrhage and none of these required transfusion or surgery.

While this seems, on the surface, to be too good to be true, a moment's thought will help us understand why this is so. Our 21 gauge needle is about the same size as the suture material which surgeons use every day in repairing damage to the abdomen; if these sutures do not cause serious problems, it is not surprising that our needle also does not. Much larger needles have been used for years for direct aortography without a serious problem with hemorrhage. Finally, our needle is actually in the patient a very short time—usually less than 5 seconds per pass—and therefore the opportunity for damage is small.

Someone is always sure to drag out that old chestnut about spreading tumor cells along a needle track. We know now how people must have felt during the heyday of Senator Joseph McCarthy; it is very hard to disprove a theory as long as people keep assuming its truth and thrusting the burden of proof on the accused. While the concept of spreading tumor cells along a needle track is intellectually attractive, it has little basis in fact. There are only a few, anecdotal case reports of this occurring in the literature while there have been several laboratory studies designed to show this phenomenon which have not been able to document its existence. We do not mean to say that this is impossible; but, if it does occur, it is exceedingly rare and should not be used as an excuse to deny patients the very real benefits of a biopsy.

UTILITY

In a large percentage of cases where a biopsy has been performed significantly useful data have been obtained. Benefits may range from verifying the benign nature of a renal cyst and thereby sparing a patient arteriography or surgery to getting an L/S ratio on amniotic fluid and thereby preventing a premature delivery. Even the patient with cancer can experience significant benefit if a biopsy is performed early. Although this early diagnosis may not change the overall outcome in these patients, it can certainly improve the quality of their remaining life by obviating the need for extensive and expensive hospital tests, and often exploratory surgery. We feel that guided biopsy will ultimately turn out to be one of the biggest contributions which ultrasound can make to better patient care. We hope that everyone who does B-mode ultrasound will do as much as they can to spread its use.

(*Irony department:* CT body scanners have been around for only a couple of years and CT-guided biopsy for even less time than that. Yet, even in this brief period of time the glamor of the CT scan is rubbing off on the biopsy procedure. Doctors who would not lend an ear to earlier descriptions of guided biopsy using ultrasound are now eagerly talking about the "new frontier" of CT-guided biopsy. Biopsy can indeed be guided by CT scanning, albeit this is a cumbersome procedure which is expensive, time-consuming and has no advantages over ultrasound. The biopsy needle is in the patient for a considerable period of time while the CT scan is being performed, yet apparently does not hurt the patient—proving, once again, what a safe procedure this is. Well, such is life. Although ultrasonographers' pride may be damaged by the attention given CT biopsy, the net effect is all to the good. Anything which promotes the acceptance of this procedure will be to the good of medicine; once the procedure is well established, people can then "rediscover" the advantages of ultrasonically guided biopsy.)

BIBLIOGRAPHY

We have lost count of the number of times we have stressed that the ideas and discussions in this book are only a starting point on the road of clinical ultrasonography. In this respect our manual does not differ from those of Alex Comfort; it is only through actual participation that you will learn to be an ultrasonographer. You have been exposed to the experience of two ultrasonographers and nothing more. We believe that if you have read and understood our message, you will have a firm foundation on which to build your own experience. Many other authors have shared their ideas in print and you will, of course, want to know what they have to say. The following bibliography should give you enough material to begin to branch out in this field. We have made no effort to compile a complete or exhaustive list of references; the books and articles cited were selected either because they are widely available or because we felt they were of particular interest, or for both reasons. Of necessity many worthwhile articles are not included, and conversely, we do not agree with the content of some that we have listed; however, all of them contain information which is of interest to anyone doing B-mode ultrasonography.

BOOKS AND MONOGRAPHS

Abdominal Echography: Ultrasound in the Diagnosis of Abdominal Conditions
by E. Barnett and P. Morley
Butterworth & Co., London, 1974

(The section on renal scanning is good but the remainder is disappointing. Scans were done with European bi-stable equipment and hence have limited applicability to American gray scale scanners.)

Fundamentals of Medical Ultrasonography
edited by G. Baum
G. P. Putnam's Sons, New York, 1973

(A big book of limited interest to abdominal ultrasonographers. The section on physics is quite good, as is the material on ophthalmologic ultrasound. The abdomen is severely short-changed.)

Seminars in Roentgenology, Vol. X, No. 4
edited by R. Brown
Grune & Stratton, Inc., New York, 1975

(The October 1975 issue of Seminars was devoted to ultrasound. Although there are scattered highlights this is overall a very disappointing work.)

Ultrasonography: Basic Principles and Clinical Applications
by R. E. Brown
Warren H. Green, Inc., St. Louis, 1975

(The strength of this text is the single authorship and, hence, the unified approach. Its weakness is that there is no gray scale. There is a discussion of other uses of ultrasound including Doppler venography.)

Cross-Section Anatomy: Computed Tomography and Ultrasound Correlation
by B. L. Carter and others
Appleton-Century-Crofts, New York, 1977

(An atlas of anatomy with both CT and ultrasound pictures.)

Diagnostic Uses of Ultrasound
by B. B. Goldberg and others
Grune & Stratton, New York, 1975

(Another general text, this book seems more dated than the copyright suggests. Over half of the text does not concern abdominal scanning.)

Diagnostic Ultrasound
by B. B. Gosink and L. F. Squire
W. B. Saunders Co., Philadelphia, 1976

(This is one of Dr. Squire's series of workbooks in diagnostic radiology and, as always, she makes learning fun. Like Dr. Leopold, Dr. Gosink shows us cross-sections upside down which is somewhat confusing. This is a fine introduction to diagnostic ultrasound but is too elementary for those working in the field.)

Diagnostic Ultrasound
edited by S. Gottlieb and M. Viamonte
American College of Radiology, 1976

(For those who think ultrasound is what the Concorde SST makes. This is too elementary for anyone actively engaged in the field.)

Abdominal Ultrasound Scanning
by H. H. Holm and others
University Park Press, Baltimore, 1976

(This little known book deserves attention. Exquisitely illustrated, its only two drawbacks are the paucity of gray scale material and the high price.)

Diagnostic Ultrasound
edited by D. L. King
C. V. Mosby Co., St. Louis, 1974

(This was among the first ultrasound texts and was one of the best. Unfortunately much of the material is now outdated but some chapters are still timely. The price is inflated.)

Atlas of Ultrasonography in Obstetrics and Gynecology
by M. Kobayashi, L. M. Hellman, and E. Cromb
Appleton-Century-Crofts, New York, 1972

(For several years this has been the classic OB text—complete with BPD and gestational sac measurements. Today we use gray scale so this venerable bi-stable atlas tends to collect dust.)

Fundamentals of Abdominal and Pelvic Ultrasonography
by G. R. Leopold and M. W. Asher
W. B. Saunders Co., Philadelphia, 1975

(Dr. Leopold orients his transverse sections as if viewed from the head which is somewhat annoying; otherwise this is a good exposition of the state of the art as of 1975. The text is particularly well-referenced and there are excellent color plates of cadaver sections. The ultrasonograms are bi-stable.)

Diagnostic Ultrasonics: Principles and Use of Instruments
by W. N. McDicken
John Wiley and Sons, Inc., New York, 1976.

(A physics book—more up-to-date than Wells'—primarily for those who dig physics.)

Recent Advances in Diagnostic Ultrasound
edited by E. Rand
Charles C Thomas, Springfield, Ill., 1971

(The title is misleading; the text is neither recent nor good. Avoid this one.)

Radiologic Clinics of North America, Vol. 13, No. 3
edited by R. C. Sanders
W. B. Saunders Co., Philadelphia, 1975

(The December 1975 issue of the Clinics is devoted to B-mode ultrasound and is the first text available which discusses gray scale. The multiple authorship makes for uneven reading but most of the contributors have done an excellent job. This is the best single text available on B-scanning, except for the one you're reading, of course.)

Ultrasound in Obstetrics and Gynecology
by R. C. Sanders
Appleton-Century-Crofts, New York, 1977

(This is hot off the press and we haven't had a chance to review it.)

Atlas of Ultrasonic Diagnosis in Obstetrics and Gynecology
by Karl-Heinz Schelensker
Publishing Sciences Group Inc., Acton, Mass., 1975

(We haven't read this one, but it is said to be a meticulously written text with beautiful, albeit bi-stable, illustrations.)

Physical Principles of Ultrasonic Diagnosis
by P. N. Wells
Academic Press, New York, 1969

(A physics book—hard going for the uninitiated and somewhat dated, this is still the classic physics text.)

Review of Ultrasound in Medical Diagnosis
by D. N. White
Ultramedison, Ontario, 1976

(This is a physics book which we have not read but which has received good reviews.)

Ultrasound in Medicine, Vols. I–III
edited by D. N. White
Plenum Press, New York, 1975–77

(Behind the impressive title lurk the proceedings of the annual meetings of the American Institute of Ultrasound in Medicine for the years beginning in 1974. This will presumably be an annual publication. These books are of limited value to the clinical ultrasonographer—there is lots of chaff and the best presentations seem to turn up in other publications. If you are going to take your ultrasound very seriously you might be interested in these as a source of some obscure ideas.)

JOURNALS

Journal of Clinical Ultrasound
John Wiley & Sons, Inc., Denver

(This publication is now five years old and seems to be thriving—it is the best single journal available on B-mode. Particularly helpful is the bimonthly reference list of current ultrasound publications.)

Radiology
The Radiologic Society of North America, Easton, Pa.

(This is primarily a radiologic journal but usually has two or three ultrasound articles a month. The ultrasound quality is uneven and the publication delay scandalous, but many worthwhile articles appear here.)

American Journal of Radiology
Charles C Thomas, Springfield, Ill.

(Although primarily a radiology journal there is usually at least one ultrasound article per month. Publication delay is not as great as with *Radiology* and the articles are, by and large, good.)

American Journal of Obstetrics and Gynecology
C. V. Mosby Co., St. Louis

(Ultrasound articles are infrequent but are often quite good.)

Ultrasound in Medicine and Biology
Pergamon Press, New York

(This journal was launched, with considerable fanfare, in 1973 but has apparently misfired: less than two full volumes have appeared in almost four years. It seems to be sputtering toward extinction.)

Medical Ultrasound
John Wiley & Sons, Inc., Denver

(This is a brand new journal and we don't know what it will be like. It is the official publication of the American Society of Ultrasound Technical Specialists.)

Reflections
American Institute of Ultrasound in Medicine, Oklahoma City

(This is not really a journal—it is the quarterly newsletter of the AIUM in slick cover. Join AIUM and you get it free.)

ARTICLES

Physics

Kossoff, G., Garrett W. J., Carpenter D. A., et al:
Principles and classification of soft tissue by gray scale echography.
Ultra. Med. Biol. 2:89 (1976)

(An excellent discussion of the theory of gray scale scanning by the group who pioneered it.)

Carlsen E. N.:
Ultrasound physics for the physician—a brief review.
J. Clin. Ultra. 3:69 (1975)

(Just what the title says.)

Kossoff, G.:
Display techniques in ultrasound pulse echo investigations. A review.
J. Clin. Ultra. 2:61 (1974)

(A very nice review of physics; more advanced than Dr. Carlsen's but quite understandable.)

Taylor, K. J. W.:
Current status of toxicity investigations.
J. Clin. Ultra. 2:149 (1974)

(Although no longer "current" the message is unchanged—no harmful effects at diagnostic intensities.)

Abdomen

Garrett, W. J., Kossoff, G., and Carpenter, D. A.:
Gray scale compound scan echography of the normal upper abdomen.
J. Clin. Ultra. 3:199 (1975)

(Gray scale pictures made with the oscilloscope–film display technique—lovely.)

Leopold, G. R.:
Gray scale ultrasonic angiography of the upper abdomen.
Radiology 117:665 (1975)

(Another demonstration of normal anatomy in gray scale—scan converter display.)

Carlsen, E. N., and Filly, R. A.:
Newer ultrasonic anatomy in the upper abdomen. (Parts I and II)
J. Clin. Ultra. 4:85 (1976)

(The anatomy isn't really new but the discussion and pictures are excellent. This is a much more pleasant method of learning anatomy than looking at an atlas.)

Sample, W. F., Gray, R. K., Poe, N. D., et al:
Nuclear imaging, tomographic nuclear imaging and gray scale ultrasound in the evaluation of the porta hepatis.
Radiology 122:773 (1977)

(A picture show; and Dr. Sample has some lovely ones.)

Skolnik, M. L., Meire, H. B., and Lecky, J. W.:
Common artifacts in ultrasound scanning.
J. Clin. Ultra. 3:273 (1975)

(Common sense stuff—if you read Chapter 5 and use your head you won't need this.)

Rasmussen, S. N., Nielsen, S. S., Bartrum, R. J., et al:
3-dimensional imaging of abdominal organs with ultrasound.
Am. J. Roentgenol. 121:883 (1974)

(Several years ago some preliminary work on computer reconstruction of serial ultrasonic sections to form a 3-dimensional image was done. It never caught on and lies fallow; however, current interest in using similar techniques for reconstructing CT scans may spill over to ultrasound and spark a revival.)

Walls, W. J., Roberts, F. F., and Templeton, A. W.:
B-scan diagnostic ultrasound in the pediatric patient.
Am. J. Roentgenol. 120:431 (1974)

(There have been many papers on pediatric ultrasound—this is one of the earliest—and they all say basically the same thing. Scanning a child is just like scanning an adult: the techniques, anatomy, and ultrasonic information are the same.)

Smith, E. H., and Holm, H. H.:
Ultrasonic scanning in radiotherapy treatment planning.
Radiology 96:433 (1970)

(There has been very little new information on the subject since this first discussion.)

Aorta

Winsberg, F., Cole-Beuglet, C., and Mulder, D. S.:
Continuous ultrasound "B" scanning of abdominal aortic aneurysms.
Am. J. Roentgenol. 121:626 (1974)

(We cite this article to introduce you to real-time B-mode scanning. Although such scanners have been available for years they are just beginning to compete with standard static image quality. Technical developments in the next few years may change this relationship.)

Retroperitoneum

Leopold, G. R.:
A review of retroperitoneal ultrasonography
J. Clin. Ultra. 1:75 (1973)

(Just what the title says.)

Smith, E. H., and Bartrum, R. J.:
Ultrasonic evaluation of pararenal masses.
J.A.M.A. 231:51 (1975)

(A picture show.)

Gallbladder

Crow, H. C., Bartrum, R. J., and Foote, S. R.:
Expanded criteria for the ultrasonic diagnosis of gallstones.
J. Clin. Ultra. 4:289 (1976)

(Unfortunately all illustrations are bi-stable but criteria for diagnosing gallstones are well described—we think!)

Arnon, S. and Rosenquist, C. J.:
Gray scale cholecystosonography: An evaluation of accuracy.
Am. J. Roentgenol. 127:817 (1976)

(Results of a study of 123 patients: ultrasound is 90 per cent accurate in detecting gallstones.)

Bartrum, R. J., Crow, H. C., and Foote, S. R.:
Ultrasonic and radiographic cholecystography.
New Eng. J. Med. 296:538 (1977)

(Our results with ultrasonic cholecystography—a prospective double-blind trial in 200 patients. Oral cholecystography is still number one but ultrasound is nearly as good.)

Leopold, G. R., Amberg, J., Gosink, B. B., et al.:
Gray scale ultrasonic cholecystography: a comparison with conventional radiographic techniques.
Radiology *121*:445 (1976)

(Documentation of the accuracy of ultrasonic cholecystography.)

Liver

Rasmussen, S. N., Holm, H. H., Kristensen, J. K., et al:
Ultrasound in the diagnosis of liver disease.
J. Clin. Ultra. *1*:220 (1973)

(A review limited to discussing bi-stable scans, this article is of interest because it describes some less known uses of ultrasound, such as liver volume determination and 3-dimensional imaging.)

Taylor, K. J. W., Carpenter, D. A., and McCready, V. R.:
Grey scale echography in the diagnosis of intrahepatic disease.
J. Clin. Ultra. *1*:284 (1973)

(An early—and realistic—discussion of gray scale and the liver.)

Taylor K. J. W., Sullivan, D., Rosenfield, A. T., et al:
Gray scale ultrasound and isotope scanning: complementary techniques for imaging the liver.
Am. J. Roentgenol. *128*:277 (1977)

(This article is similar to many others by Dr. Taylor. He is able to achieve a diagnostic accuracy in the liver which few other groups can match.)

Pancreas

Sokoloff, J., Gosink, B. B., Leopold, G. R., et al:
Pitfalls in the echographic evaluation of pancreatic disease.
J. Clin. Ultra. 2:321 (1974)

(Pictures are bi-stable and upside down but the discussion is good.)

Walls, W. J., Gonzalez, G., Martin, N. L., et al:
B-scan ultrasound evaluation of the pancreas. Advantages and accuracy compared to other diagnostic techniques.
Radiology *114*:127 (1975)

(A comparison study with actual numbers rather than just opinions.)

Doust B. D., and Pearce, J. D.:
Gray scale ultrasonic properties of the normal and inflamed pancreas.
Radiology *120*:653 (1976)

(Worthwhile review of gray scale findings in 52 patients with pancreatitis.)

Haber, K., Freimais, A. K., and Asher, W. M.:
Demonstration and dimensional analysis of the normal pancreas with gray scale echography.
Am. J. Roentgenol. *126*:624 (1976)

(This article lists measurements for the "normal" pancreas: this is fine if you like that sort of thing. We don't. A few years ago we reviewed 600 pancreatic scans done with bi-stable technique, and could not find any "measurement" which would reliably separate normal from abnormal glands. We feel this is a subjective determination—the abnormal pancreas looks too big for its surroundings.)

Hancke, S.:
Ultrasonic scanning of the pancreas.
J. Clin. Ultra. *4*:223 (1976)

(A thorough review of the subject. Illustrations are bi-stable but the principles are universal.)

Ghorashi, B. and Rector, W. R.:
Gray scale sonographic anatomy of the pancreas.
J. Clin. Ultra. 5:25 (1977)

(Nice pictures, exhaustive discussion.)

Spleen

Koga, T. and Morikawa, Y.:
Ultrasonographic determination of splenic size and its clinical usefulness in various liver diseases.
Radiology *115*:157 (1975)

(Tells you how to measure spleen size — much ado about nothing.)

Asher, W. M., Parvin, S., Virgilio, R. W., et al:
Echographic evaluation of splenic injury after blunt trauma.
Radiology *118*:411 (1976)

(While we do not agree with the authors' conclusion that "ultrasound is considered to be an excellent screening procedure for suspected splenic rupture," this is as good a description as exists of the ultrasonic appearance of the spleen.)

Kidney

Green, W. M. and King, D. L.:
Diagnostic ultrasound of the urinary tract.
J. Clin. Ultra. *4*:55 (1976)

(An up-to-date review.)

Green, W. M., King, D. L., and Casarella, W. J.:
A reappraisal of sonolucent renal masses.
Radiology *121*:163 (1976)

(The authors wisely caution against relying too heavily on any single study in evaluating renal masses — this article is a must for those who do renal scans.)

Sanders, R. C., and Jeck, D. L.:
B-scan ultrasound in the evaluation of renal failure.
Radiology *119*:199 (1976)

(Although pictures are bi-stable the discussion applies to gray scale as well.)

Schneider, M., Becker, J. A., Staiano, S., et al:
Sonographic-radiographic correlation of renal and peri-renal infections.
Am. J. Roentgenol. *127*:1007 (1976)

(As we'd expect, ultrasound is mainly of value when there is a peri-renal abscess.)

Bartrum, R. J., Smith, E. H., D'Orsi, C. J., et al:
Evaluation of renal transplants with ultrasound.
Radiology *118*:405 (1976)

(Title is self-explanatory: if you don't examine transplant patients you won't need this.)

Pelvis

Cochrane, W. J. and Thomas, M. A.:
Ultrasound diagnosis of gnyecologic pelvic masses.
Radiology *110*:649 (1974)

(Results in a large series of patients.)

Watanabe, H., Igari, D., Tanakashi, Y., et al:
Development and applications of new equipment for transrectal ultrasonography.
J. Clin. Ultra. *2*:91 (1974)

(An article on an unusual use for ultrasound.)

Haller, J. O., Schneider, M., Kassner, E. G., et al.:
Ultrasonography in pediatric gynecology and obstetrics.
Am. J. Roentgenol. *128*:423 (1977)

(There is no difference in scanning the young and adult pelvis — same technique, diseases, and results.)

Pregnancy

King, D. L.:
Placental ultrasonography.
J. Clin. Ultra. *1*:21 (1973)

(Although not a new reference, there is little this leaves unsaid.)

Winsberg, F.:
Echographic changes of placental aging.
J. Clin. Ultra. *1*:52 (1973)

(Although many of us take issue with the conclusion that the parabolic mirror-rotating transducer real-time scanner is the best way to scan the placenta, we all agree on the concept of placental aging.)

Thompson, H. E.:
Ultrasonic diagnostic procedures in obstetrics and gynecology.
J. Clin. Ultra. *1*:160 (1973)

(A basic article, complete with graphs for BPD, gestational sac, and fetal thorax measurements.)

Levi, S., and Smets, P.:
Intra-uterine growth studied by ultrasonic bi-parietal measurements.
Acta Obstet. Gynec. Scand. 52:193 (1973)

(There are several large studies giving the derivation of gestational age tables; this is our favorite and includes mean as well as percentile growth tables.)

Wiener, S. N., Flynn, M. J., Kennedy A. W., et al:
A composite curve of ultrasonic biparietal diameters for estimating gestational age.
Radiology *122*:781 (1977)

(Those who can't decide between the many BPD charts will want this mathematical synthesis of available data into one "composite" curve. Unfortunately the data are presented as a graph rather than a table but the latter is probably available from the authors.)

Barlotucci, L.:
Biparietal diameter of the skull and fetal weight in the second trimester: An allometric relationship.
Am. J. Obstet. Gynec. *122*:439 (1975)

(There are scores of papers proposing methods of increasing the accuracy of gestational dating — this is a typical example. We feel that such efforts are much ado about nothing as they seem to ignore a major fact of life: there are normal inherent variations in all biologic processes including fetal development. Try as we might, it is impossible to force all fetuses to develop according to a predetermined schedule.)

Scheer, K.:
Ultrasound in twin gestations.
J. Clin. Ultra. 2:197 (1974)

(The twins ignore each other. Both heads grow at the same rate and the BPD charts for single gestations can be used with no corrections.)

Lawson, T. L., Albarelli, J. N., Greenhouse, S. W., et al:
Gray scale measurement of biparietal diameter.
J. Clin. Ultra. 5:17 (1977)

(If you are going to use gray scale to measure BPD's, this will give you comfort. We still prefer bi-stable.)

Kurjak, A., Ceuck, S., and Breger, B.:
Prediction of maturity in first trimester of pregnancy by ultrasonic measurement of fetal crown rump length.
J. Clin. Ultra. 4:83 (1976)

(We think this is unnecessary but if you like measuring things here is another graph.)

Queenan, J. T., Kubarych, S. F., Cook, L. N., et al.:
Diagnostic ultrasound for detection of intrauterine growth retardation.
Am. J. Obstet. Gynec. *124*:865 (1976)

(We are not convinced that IUGR can be diagnosed by ultrasound. This paper and the discussion which follows examine the problems.)

Ghorashi, B., and Gottesfeld, K. R.:
Recognition of the hydropic fetus by gray scale ultrasound.
J. Clin. Ultra. 4:193 (1976)

(Nice pictures, good discussion of this process.)

Levi, S.:
Ultrasonic assessment of the high rate of human multiple pregnancy in the first trimester.
J. Clin. Ultra. 4:3 (1976)

(It seems there are more twins in the first trimester than are delivered. Where do the extra babies go? Several explanations suggest themselves. Fascinating reading.)

Phillips, J. F., Goodwin, D. W., Thomason, S. B., et al:
The volume of the uterus in normal and abnormal pregnancy.
J Clin Ultrasound 5:107 (1977)

(Diagnosing oligo- or polyhydramnios is a very subjective procedure at best. Most of the time it is better not to comment on the amount of amniotic fluid. This paper discusses a method of making this a more objective determination.)

Miscellaneous

Skolnick, M. L. and Royal, D. B.:
A simple and inexpensive water bath adapting a contact scanner for thyroid and testicular imaging.
J. Clin. Ultra. 3:225 (1975)

(How to build an open water bath for peanuts.)

Crocker, E. F., McLaughlin, A. F., Kossoff, G., et al:
The gray scale echographic appearance of thyroid malignancy.
J. Clin. Ultra. 2:305 (1974)

(There is some hope that ultrasound will ultimately be able to distinguish benign from malignant thyroid nodules.)

Rosen, I. B., Walfish, P. G., and Miskin, M.:
The use of B-mode ultrasonography in changing indications for thyroid operations.
Surg. Gynec. Obstet. 139:193 (1974)

(While we don't share the authors' confidence in making highly specific diagnoses, this is one of the largest reported series of thyroid scans.)

Chilcote, W. S.:
Gray-scale ultrasonography of the thyroid.
Radiology 120:381 (1976)

(Ultrasound can distinguish cystic from solid but not benign from malignant.)

Baum, G.:
Ultrasound mammography.
Radiology 122:199 (1977)

(This is the best summary of this subject in our opinion—it strikes a realistic viewpoint.)

Kobayashi, T.:
Gray-scale echography for breast cancer.
Radiology 122:207 (1977)

(Be sure to read Dr. G. Baum's paper after you read this.)

Miskin, M. and Baum, J.:
B-mode ultrasonic examination of the testes.
J. Clin. Ultra. 2:307 (1974)

(One of the few articles on this topic.)

Shawker, T. H.:
B-mode ultrasonic evaluation of scrotal swellings.
Radiology 118:417 (1976)

(Similar to the preceding article.)

Doust, B. D., Baum, J. K., Maklad, N. F., et al:
Ultrasonic evaluation of pleural opacities.
Radiology 114:135 (1975)

(A complete discourse on finding pleural effusions with ultrasound.)

Goldberg, B. B.:
Ultrasonic evaluation of superficial masses.
J. Clin. Ultra. 3:91 (1975)

(Ultrasound·is pretty good at telling if such masses are cystic or solid.)

Neiman, H. L., Phillips, J. F., Jaques, D. A., et al:
Ultrasound of the parotid gland.
J. Clin. Ultra. 4:11 (1976)

(Nothing earthshaking—ultrasound can differentiate cystic from solid masses.)

Sigel, B., Popky, G. L., Wagner, D. K., et al:
A Doppler ultrasound method for diagnosing lower extremity venous disease.
Surg. Gynec. Obstet. 126:339 (1968)

(As promised, a reference on the technique of Doppler venography. This procedure has not achieved wide popularity.)

Biopsy

Holm, H. H., Pedersen, J. F., Kristensen, J. K., et al:
Ultrasonically guided percutaneous puncture.
Rad. Clin. North Amer. 13:493 (1975)

(Dr. Holm's group were pioneers in this procedure and have many years of experience with it. This excellent article summarizes their work.)

Goldberg, B. B. and Pollack, H. H.:
Ultrasonic aspiration biopsy techniques.
J. Clin. Ultra. 4:141 (1976)

(A review of the subject—everything you always wanted to know, and more.)

INDEX